Adolescent Health

ISSUES

Volume 70

Editor

Craig Donnellan

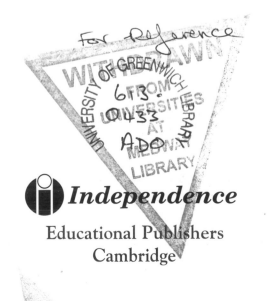

Independence

Educational Publishers
Cambridge

First published by Independence
PO Box 295
Cambridge CB1 3XP
England

British Library Cataloguing in Publication Data
Adolescent Health – (Issues Series)
I. Donnellan, Craig II. Series
613'.0433

ISBN 1 86168 252 2

Printed in Great Britain
MWL Print Group Ltd

Typeset by
Claire Boyd

Cover
The illustration on the front cover is by
Pumpkin House.

CONTENTS

Chapter One: Overview

Chapter Two: Issues in Adolescent Health

Introduction

Adolescent Health is the seventieth volume in the **Issues** series. The aim of this series is to offer up-to-date information about important issues in our world.

Adolescent Health examines the key health issues affecting young people.

The information comes from a wide variety of sources and includes:
Government reports and statistics
Newspaper reports and features
Magazine articles and surveys
Web site material
Literature from lobby groups
and charitable organisations.

It is hoped that, as you read about the many aspects of the issues explored in this book, you will critically evaluate the information presented. It is important that you decide whether you are being presented with facts or opinions. Does the writer give a biased or an unbiased report? If an opinion is being expressed, do you agree with the writer?

Adolescent Health offers a useful starting-point for those who need convenient access to information about the many issues involved. However, it is only a starting-point. At the back of the book is a list of organisations which you may want to contact for further information.

*****

Adolescents' general health and wellbeing

General health and wellbeing

Adolescence is a period of greatly enhanced awareness of and attention to physical status and wellbeing. This period is traditionally viewed as a time of optimal health with low levels of morbidity and chronic disease. Indeed, from previous experience in the United States, the vast majority of middle-school students (93%) have reported being in good, very good or excellent health. Nevertheless, suicide, depression, other mental health conditions, AIDS and other adolescent-focused risks threaten this notion of prevailing good health for adolescence. This notion is related to the overall utilisation of health services and exposure to health risks. The concept of measuring adolescent health through standardised self-report is well established. Thus, a global measure of general health was included in the HBSC survey and in the international comparative analyses to measure the perceived impact of health risks on this population.

Feeling healthy

General health status was assessed by a single question that asked: 'How healthy do you think you are?' Response choices were: 'very healthy', 'quite healthy' (or in some questionnaires, 'somewhat healthy'), or 'not very healthy'. The first two responses were combined to derive a variable of feeling healthy, in contrast to not very healthy.

As in the last *Health Behaviour in School-Aged Children* (HBSC) survey, most students in the 1997/ 1998 survey consider themselves healthy (total 91.8%, range 81.2% to 98.0%). By a small but consistent difference, a higher percentage of males (93.7%) than females (90.0%)

By Peter Scheidt, Mary D. Overpeck, Wendy Wyatt and Anna Aszmann

report feeling very healthy; and this pattern is consistent for all countries and regions. The youngest girls have the highest levels of feeling healthy (93.0%), and the percentage decreases for each subsequent age group (from 91.2% to 87.4%). Percentages of 11- and 13-year-old boys who feel healthy are similar (over 95%), with slight decreases for 15-year-old boys (93.6%). The same trend is seen among all participating countries and for both genders, though the differences between age groups are not as great as those between genders.

As reported from the last survey, young people in Sweden report the highest rates of feeling healthy (98.0%), but rates for Finnish young

people, previously in the middle, are now comparable. Least positive about their health are the young people of four countries in central and eastern Europe (84.2–88.8%) and the Russian Federation (81.2%). Students from the United States along with those in Wales, Estonia, and Northern Ireland, are relatively negative about their health.

Feeling happy

Assessments of how students feel about life in general, whether they feel low (have negative affect) or lonely, although not a direct measure of health, are included for correlation with symptoms and health outcome as factors that often affect or are affected by health, and as indicators of mental health.

How the students feel in general was assessed by asking: 'In general, how do you feel about your life at present?' Responses included: 'I feel very happy', 'I feel quite happy', 'I

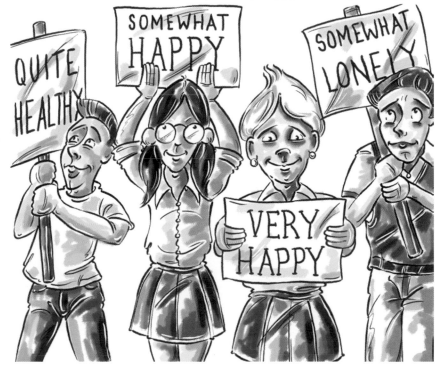

don't feel very happy' and 'I am not happy at all'. The first two and the last two were combined to derive measures of feeling happy and not feeling happy, respectively.

The vast majority of students report feeling happy (85.2%, 62.2% and 94.1% of 11-, 13- and 15-year-olds, respectively), although the percentages are not as high as those for feeling healthy. As with feeling healthy, boys are more positive overall than girls by 5%, and positive responses decrease as the students advance in age. The least happy students are those from Israel (62.2%). Interestingly, students from central and eastern Europe and the Russian Federation are as negative about their emotional state as their health. The most positive feelings are reported from Scandinavia (Sweden (94.1%), Norway (93.7%) and Denmark (93.6%)), followed by other northern European countries: Switzerland (93.3%), Austria (92.8%), England (92.3%), Flemish-speaking Belgium (92.1%), Finland (91.4%), Northern Ireland (90.0%), Germany (89.3%) and Ireland (89.2).

Feeling lonely

Feeling lonely was assessed by a single direct question: 'Do you ever feel lonely?' responses included: 'No', 'Yes, sometimes', 'Yes, rather often', 'Yes, very often'. The last two responses were combined to show the rate of students who report often feeling lonely.

Though most students do not report feeling lonely, such feelings are still common, exceeding 10% in all but four countries. As with negative feelings about life and feeling low, feeling lonely occurs more often in girls than boys at all ages and increases as girls grow older. For boys, loneliness is substantially lower and remains the same through this period of adolescence. Two countries, Portugal and Israel, report loneliness rates much higher than those in all other countries.

Feeling low

Depressive affect was assessed by including in the multipart question about symptoms: 'In the past 6 months, how often have you had the following: feeling low.' Responses included: 'Rarely or never', 'About

once every month', 'About once every week', 'More than once a week' and 'About every day'. For this comparison, the last three responses were combined to derive a rate of reporting low feelings at least once a week.

The overall percentage of students feeling low on a weekly basis is relatively high, averaging over 25%, with the students of all but one country exceeding 10%. The negative affect is higher for girls than boys for all ages, and increases with age. In contrast, the relatively lower frequency of negative affect for boys remains stable at about 20% for the three age groups. The highest rates of feeling low (over 40%) are found in Greece, Israel, and Hungary, with the United States relatively close at 38%.

Feeling tired

Feelings of excessive tiredness or sleepiness do not contribute to a sense of wellbeing. Although not in general a problem for preadolescents, excessive daytime sleepiness has long been observed in adolescence. HBSC

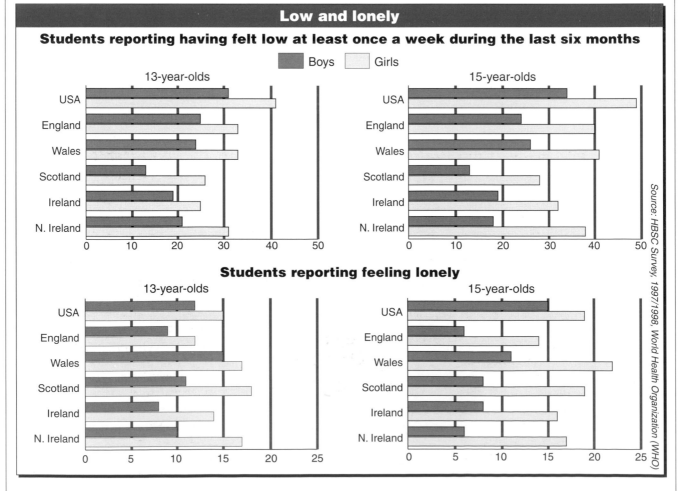

Source: HBSC Survey, 1997/1998, World Health Organization (WHO)

has previously documented a high frequency of morning tiredness associated with watching television, using psychoactive substances and decreasing physical activity. Feeling tired or sleepy in the morning can be an indication of increased demand for sleep, insufficient rest or pathological disturbance, such as depression. Sleep deprivation is an increasing fact of modern life, and progressive reductions in sleep time associated with sleepiness have been documented as children move into adolescence. Feeling tired in adolescence, however, also increases with physical and endocrinological maturation in the absence of any change in total nocturnal sleep time. In the United States and Israel, over the past several years, reports have suggested that the biological rhythms of adolescents are not suited to early morning waking. These observations have led to moving school starting times to later in the morning for high-school students in some districts. The frequency of perceived morning fatigue can be useful as an indicator of differences in socio-cultural patterns, a basis for pro-gramme changes and as a marker for problems such as depression or chronic illness.

Morning tiredness was assessed with a question, 'How often do you feel tired when you go to school in the morning?' Responses included: 'Rarely or never', 'Occasionally (less than once a week)', '1 to 3 times a week' and '4 or more times a week'. The analysis focused on the frequency of feeling tired most of the time: 4 or more times a week.

As also noted from other studies, morning tiredness is reported frequently in most of the countries participating in HBSC. The average rate of morning sleepiness on a weekly basis is 40%, with a range of 16-60%. An average of 22% of students report fatigue most days of the week, with a range of about 7-45%. In contrast to perception of health and other symptoms, boys feel more morning sleepiness than girls in all three age groups. Overall and for most countries, the percentage of students feeling tired increases with age for both boys and girls. Proportions of respondents reporting feeling tired in the morning at least 4 times a week are highest in Norwegian students followed by those from Finland and the United States. Given the relatively low frequency of other symptoms for Norwegian students, the figures for morning sleepiness may be related to the time of year of survey administration (December), or possibly the high latitude, school schedules or other factors.

■ The above information is an extract from *Health and Health Behaviour among Young People* which is produced by the World Health Organization Regional Office for Europe. The series *Health Policy for Children and Adolescents* (HEPCA) is a WHO publication series mainly based on results of the international survey *Health Behaviour in School-aged Children* (HBSC) and on other relevant international studies.

■ For further information, please contact: WHO Regional Office for Europe, 8 Scherfigsvej, DK-2100 Copenhagen, Denmark. Tel: +45 39 17 17 17. Fax: +45 39 17 18 18. E-mail: postmaster@who.dk Web site: www.who.dk

© *World Health Organization*

Young people have major health needs

Information from *Bridging the Gaps: Health Care for Adolescents*, produced by the Royal College of Paediatrics and Child Health

Adolescents make up a significant proportion of the population; in the UK, along with most developed countries, young people between the ages of 10 and 20 account for 13-15% of the total. Projections suggest that the adolescent population will grow by 8.5% between 1998 and 2011.

Mortality among adolescents, in contrast to almost all other age groups, did not fall during the second half of the twentieth century. The main causes of mortality in this age group are accidents and self-harm. Adolescents' health needs appear to be greater than those of children in the middle childhood (from 5 to 12 years) or of young adults. Morbidity mainly arises from chronic illness and mental health problems; Child and Adolescent Mental Health Services (CAMHS) are often both seen as, and are, the poor relation of

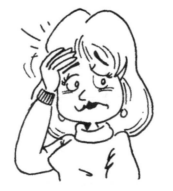

other services in terms of resources. This in spite of the fact that long-term morbidity and mortality among young people with mental health problems is among the highest of any group of patients. The peak age of onset of type 1 diabetes is during adolescence and its control is poorer than at any other age. The main concerns of young people in relation to health are focused on issues of immediacy that impact on their relations with peers and include problems with skin, weight, appearance, emotions and sexual health including contraception. Young people whose childhood or adolescent illness has impacted significantly on their appearance or expectations for sexual and reproductive function face particularly intense problems as they approach adulthood.

Attendances for health care by young people aged 12 to 19 years are about half those of the traditional 'child' population aged 0 to 14 years but their use of hospital beds increases during adolescence, particularly in females and without inclusion of obstetric admissions. Nearly all have seen a GP within the previous twelve months, though there is evidence that their consultations are shorter than average; many will have seen other health professionals. They report concerns about how services are currently provided. Adolescents' health and better ways to meet their physical and mental health needs are matters of national and international concern. The brief of this report was addressed succinctly in the USA context over 20 years ago by Charles Irwin, who reached very similar conclusions to those we reach. Nearly a decade ago the President of the Society for Adolescent Health in her presidential address emphasised the importance of adolescent health practitioners recognising their role in advocacy for, rather than didactic interaction with, young people.

Adolescence is a developmental phase of significant positive change and maturation and is by no means universally problematic. Nevertheless because of the rapid emotional, social and psychological changes occurring during adolescence, together with pubertal changes in growth and strength, a number of problems may become apparent which may earlier have been 'masked'. Thus, acting out behaviours tend to be contained during primary school years but become problematic during adolescence especially in boys, while affective disorders may similarly become apparent in adolescence, particularly among girls. A young person who is being 'looked after' and therefore, by definition, experiencing significant 'disconnectedness' with family is associated with dramatically higher prevalence of mental health disorder, teenage pregnancy and involvement in crime.

Young people are not a homogeneous group but have diverse special needs associated, for example, with gender, ethnicity, social and educational disadvantage, family breakdown and sexual orientation. A significantly larger proportion of people among the minority ethnic groups in the UK is under 20 than in the host population, particularly among the Bangladeshi and Pakistani groups. These young people have particular health needs associated with their increased risk of certain health problems, and because they are over-represented among families who suffer socio-economic and health disadvantage.

It is clearly important that young people are nurtured so that they may become healthy adults and contributors to society. This is increasingly important for sound economic reasons in an ageing society. The high rates of sexually transmitted infections among young people, particularly teenage girls, are a significant cause of physical health problems and the recent rise of suicide among young men gives grave concern for psychological health. There is strong and growing evidence for the fundamental inter-relationship between physical, mental and social health. Problems in adolescence in any of these areas indicate the likelihood of long-term adverse health and social consequences. The fact that the UK has the highest rate of teenage pregnancy in western Europe is one instance of the way that many of our young people will start their adult lives at significant disadvantage.

There is evidence that patterns of health behaviours established in adolescence are maintained through adult life (e.g. smoking , substance abuse, eating disorders, physical activity, obesity and sexual risk taking). Contextual factors associated with higher risks of unhealthy behaviours in adolescence and higher risks to health, such as living in relative poverty, poor parenting, family breakdown and being looked after by the local authority are often present in the childhood years.

■ The above information is an extract from *Bridging the Gaps: Health Care for Adolescents*, produced by the Royal College of Paediatrics and Child Health – for more information and a full list of references visit their web site at www.rcpch.ac.uk/news/index.html

© Royal College of Paediatrics and Child Health

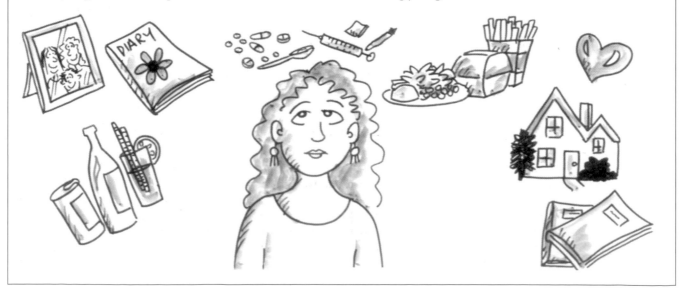

Physical activity and youth

Information from the World Health Organization

- Regular physical activity provides young people with important physical, mental and social health benefits. Regular practice of physical activity helps children and young people to build and maintain healthy bones, muscles and joints, helps control body weight, helps reduce fat and develop efficient function of the heart and lungs. It contributes to the development of movement and co-ordination and helps prevent and control feelings of anxiety and depression.

- Play, games and other physical activities give young people opportunities for self-expression, building self-confidence, feelings of achievement, social inter-action and integration. These positive effects also help counter-act the risks and harm caused by the demanding, competitive, stressful and sedentary way of life that is so common in young people's lives today. Involvement in properly guided physical activity and sports can also foster the adoption of other healthy behaviour including avoidance of tobacco, alcohol and drug use and violent behaviour. It can also foster healthy diet, adequate rest and better safety practices.

- Some studies show that among adolescents, the more often they participate in physical activity, the less likely they are to use tobacco. It has also been found that children who are more physically active showed higher academic performance. Team games and play promote positive social integration and facilitate the development of social skills in young children.

- Patterns of physical activity acquired during childhood and adolescence are more likely to be maintained throughout the life span, thus providing the basis for active and healthy life. On the other hand, unhealthy lifestyles

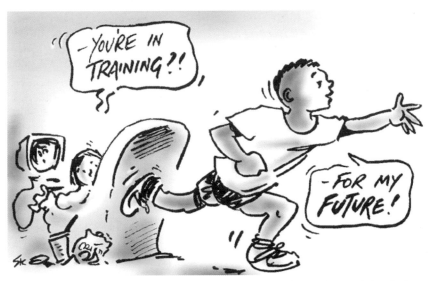

– including sedentary lifestyle, poor diet and substance abuse – adopted at a young age are likely to persist in adulthood.

- Physical activity levels are decreasing among young people in countries around the world, especially in poor urban areas. It is estimated that less than one-third of young people are sufficiently active to benefit their present and future health and well-being.

- Physical education and other school-based physical activities are also decreasing. Only a few countries offer at least two hours per week of physical education in both primary and secondary schools. These negative trends are likely to continue, even worsen and spread to an increasing number of countries.

- This decline is largely due to increasingly common sedentary ways of life. For example fewer children walk or cycle to school and excessive time is devoted to watching television, playing computer games, and using computers – very often at the expense of time and opportunities for physical activity and sports.

- Many factors prevent young people from being regularly physically active: lack of time and motivation, insufficient support and guidance from adults, feelings of embarrassment or incom-petence, lack of safe facilities and locales for physical activity, and simple ignorance of the benefits of physical activity.

- Schools present unique opportu-nities to provide time, facilities and guidance for physical activity for young people. Schools have the mandate and responsibility for enhancing all aspects of growth and development for children and young people. In most countries, through physical education programmes, schools offer the only systematic opportunity for young people to take part in and learn about physical activity.

- Ample participation in play, games and other physical activities, both in school and during free time, is essential for the healthy development of every young person. Access to safe places, opportunities and time, and good examples from teachers, parents and friends are all part of ensuring that children and young people move for health.

■ The above information is from the World Health Organization's web site which can be found at www.who.int

© World Health Organization (WHO)

Young adults

Information from Elsevier Ltd.

Adolescence may be defined as the process of growing up. The age span is variable as young people mature at different ages and speeds. The World Health Organization puts the ages between 11 and 21.

As well as the profound physical and emotional maturational changes that occur, adolescence is also a time of seeking independence, of risk-taking to 'imitate' adult behaviour and of establishing a personal identity. Family structure and the level of its support, peer group and educational environment influence adolescent behaviour. Most young people traverse adolescence without problems. If difficulties do arise, then those of early adolescence are primarily associated with physical and developmental changes, and those in late adolescence with identity change.

In order to establish personal identity young people may search for their cultural roots at this time, or for their biological parents if adopted. The question of sexual orientation may arise with the ensuing struggle to recognise and 'come out'. Many young people begin to question the fundamental values of parents and other adults, and develop a critical awareness of the world around and its social injustices. Disabled or chronically ill young people may become increasingly aware of how

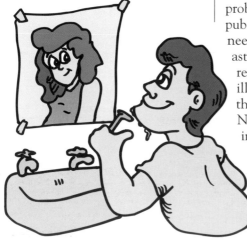

their condition impacts on their lives, which may lead to feelings of aggression, depression or even suicide. Those from ethnic minority groups may become aware of unequal opportunities, and the impact of racism. Social changes on leaving school may range from further education, to financial independence or to unemployment. Homelessness and poverty may contribute to depression and low self-esteem.

The struggle to become independent is often too threatening to accomplish alone, so many adolescents choose to go through the process in the same way as their peer group with all its pressures.

Health needs

Young people's health needs are diverse and are affected by their gender, culture, ethnic group and sexual orientation. In planning services for their needs we must take account of their physical, mental and sexual health within the context of social issues and legal rights. Confidentiality is a key issue identified by young people whatever their needs.

Physical health problems of adolescence

The physical health problems specific to adolescence fall into three main groups: disorders of puberty, diseases of adolescence (e.g. acne, bone tumours, anorexia nervosa) and problems of chronic disease during puberty associated with changing needs and poor compliance (e.g. asthma, diabetes, cystic fibrosis, renal failure). The incidence of illness in this age group is lower than that at any other time in life. Nevertheless there has been an increase in self-reported illness in the last decade (Department of Health 1994). The General Household Survey suggests adolescents visit their GP three to four times a year, mainly for respiratory tract

disease, but also for skin disorders, allergies, injuries and contraception (Churchill et al 1997).

Adolescents are concerned about a wide range of health and environmental issues, feel responsible for their own health and acknowledge that good health is mainly due to sensible living. Even though the majority consider themselves to be healthy, evidence suggests that they are at increasing risk from the harmful effects of smoking, alcohol consumption, using drugs and unsafe sex (Coleman 1997). Many of the accidents that occur in this age group are the result of risk-taking behaviour, for example excess alcohol consumption and driving, dangerous sports or not wearing protective clothing

Nutrition

There are increased nutritional requirements in adolescence for iron (for muscle mass and blood volume in males and for menstrual loss in females), calcium (for skeletal growth) and zinc (for adequate sexual maturation). Dietary status is an important part of health evaluation in adolescence .

Mortality rates

Death rates in young people are highest in the 15-19-year age group. The major causes are shown in the graph opposite.

Hospital admissions

In early adolescence admission rates are divided fairly evenly between general paediatrics, general surgery, ENT and trauma and orthopaedics. By around 16 years less than 1% are admitted for general paediatrics. Twenty-four per cent of girls are admitted for gynaecological reasons, mainly termination of pregnancy (Henderson et al 1993). Forty per cent of young men are admitted for trauma and head injuries. Self-poisoning is common in older teenage girls (Kerfoot 1996).

Social and mental health issues

Social and mental health issues are intricately entwined. The Mental Health Foundation (1999) estimates that 20% of children and adolescents are experiencing significant psychological problems. Social issues, such as homelessness and poverty, are relevant. There are individual and family factors. Three risk factors predict emotional problems for 8%, but four risk factors predict problems for 20%. Adolescents who have been sexually abused become more aware of the significance of their trauma after puberty. Self-harm and drug use became more prevalent, and either may be considered coping strategies (Herman 1998). Other traumas include bullying, changing family structure and bereavements. The Trent Lifestyle Survey reported that 8% of young people in 1994 did not feel good about any of the following: their health, the future, how they looked, what happened at home, schoolwork or friendships. Nine per cent stated there was no one to talk over problems with (Roberts et al 1995).

Mental health issues may be expressed as:

■ Drug use.
■ Self-harm and suicide.
■ Depression.
■ Truancy and offending behaviour.

Alcohol

Under-age drinking and problems associated with it are increasing in the UK. Surveys show that children drink alcohol earlier, and by their teens, drinking is a regular part of their lives. Between 92% and 98% of 15-years-olds have tried alcohol (Miller & Plant 1996, Gabhain & Francois 2000). Up to 9% of 11-year-old girls and up to 12% of 11-year-old boys have tried alcohol (Gabhain & Francois 2000). Goddard (1997) reports that more than 50% of 15-year-olds drank alcohol the previous week. Girls drank on average 7 units and boys 9.7 units. Home is the major source of the alcohol, but 5.5% of year 10s buy it from a supermarket and 23% buy it from an off-licence (Balding 1996). McKeganey (1996) reports

Children are more likely to smoke if parents and siblings do. Friends may influence them. It helps them feel independent and more attractive

more than 50% of 14-year-olds saying they have been drunk. This fits in with the World Health Organization study (Gabhain & Francois 2000) that reports between 53% and 72% of 15-year-old boys in the UK have been drunk at least twice, and 10% of 11-year-old boys. The way alcohol is used at home influences the development of drinking behaviour as young people mature. Young inexperienced drinkers have a lower tolerance to alcohol and even small amounts of alcohol significantly lower their judgement and control. One would expect drinking to be associated with unwanted sex, unprotected sex and violence.

The Confiscation of Alcohol (Young Persons) Act 1997 permits police to remove alcohol if the person is considered to be under 18 years and in a public place (Swade 1997).

Smoking

The health hazards of smoking are well recognised. The younger chil-

dren are when they begin smoking, the more likely they are to die from it as adults. Children starting to smoke at the age of 15 years are three times more likely to die from smoking than adults starting in their mid twenties (Doll & Peto 1981).

The prevalence of smoking in children aged 11-15 years has increased from 8% in 1988 to 13% in 1996. This is higher in girls, having increased from 9% to 15% (Thomas et al 1998). Eighty-two per cent of adult smokers began when they were teenagers. Is smoking a paediatric disease?

Children are more likely to smoke if parents and siblings do. Friends may influence them. It helps them feel independent and more attractive. They do not consider that the risks of smoking apply to them (Sutton 1998). There is an association with poverty, use of alcohol and drugs and educational under-achievement (McKee 1999).

Seventy per cent of children buy cigarettes from shops; 33% use vending machines. Ninety-six per cent of school children report seeing cigarette advertising in the last 6 months. Children smoke brands that are heavily advertised. Fifty per cent consider they have seen advertising on the television in the last 6 months – there has been none for 33 years (Jarvis 1997).

The UK government aims to reduce smoking in 11- 15-year-olds

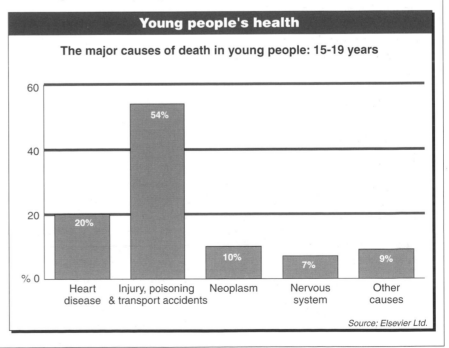

Young people's health

The major causes of death in young people: 15-19 years

Source: Elsevier Ltd.

from 13% to 11% by 2005, and to 9% by 2010. The policy is aimed at reducing access to cigarettes and making smoking less desirable in this age group (*Smoking Kills* – A White Paper on Tobacco 1998). It is a worthy aim, but innovative methods on changing young people's attitudes need evaluation.

Illegal drug use

Britain has the highest use of illicit drugs in the European Union (European Drugs Monitoring Centre 1998). McKee (1999) links this to educational under-achievement, poverty and family life with parents working the longest hours in Europe. The Police Research Group reported in August 1998 that heroin was flooding the market and being sold for £10 in areas where it had not appeared before. The majority of users are in socially deprived areas, but increasing numbers have an affluent background (Evans 1998).

Many drugs are illegal (Misuse of Drugs Act 1971), and there are penalties for being in possession or for intending to supply them.

■ The above information is from pages 381-386 from Polnay: *Community Paediatrics*, 3rd Ed.
© 2002 Elsevier Ltd.

The state of young people's health in the EU

Executive summary

As part of the series of reports on the state of health in the European Union drawn up by the European Commission, this report focuses on the health status of young people (ages 15 to 24).

Health and well-being in this age group have rarely been addressed in EU-wide comparative studies. National health information systems such as vital statistics provide valuable information, but data on aspects of health relevant to young people are not easily available. And yet, not only childhood, but also – and to a greater extent than is generally appreciated – the transition from childhood to adulthood is a crucial period during which the foundations are laid for health in future life, within the parameters of the individual's family background and economic, social, cultural and educational circumstances. There-fore, it is essential to give considera-tion not only to mortality, morbidity and lifestyles, but also more generally to well-being, functional capacity and quality of life.

The limited information that is available reveals the following general trends:

■ There is marked diversity within the European Union in terms of both the status of young people's health and health trends.

■ The majority of young people enjoy good health, and the trends from the mid-1980s to the mid-1990s suggest that the situation is likely to further improve in the future. In 1997, life expectancy at age 15 was 60.3 years for males and 66.4 years for females (years of life remaining) – an increase of two years over the last 10 years. However, some chronic condi-tions – such as asthma, allergic disorders, diabetes and obesity – are increasing.

■ A considerable proportion of young people suffer from poverty, family breakdown, lack of social support and of educational or professional challenges, or from low quality of food, all factors which may impede healthy growth and development. The marked differences both between

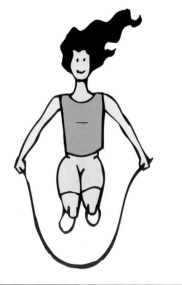

and within the Member States in social and cultural determinants of health are bound to lead to increasing inequalities in young people's health between popula-tion subgroups and countries. The following more specific results were found:

■ Each year about 30,500 lives are lost in the age range 15 to 24 in EU Member States. Premature death is more common in males (23,000) than in females (7,500). Traffic accidents are the biggest killer (about 10,000 males, 2,000 females), whilst suicides account for one in ten premature deaths.

■ Most young people regard their own health as good. However, about one-quarter suffer regularly from psychosomatic symptoms, and one in ten reports a disability that limits daily functioning (e.g. musculo-skeletal disorders).

■ Only a rough indication can be drawn of mental health trends; in the 15-24 age group, almost 10% seem to experience clinically recognisable depressive symp-toms, whereas – on the basis of the scarce data available – it is estimated that the overall pre-valence of mental disorders in adolescence is in the region of 15 to 20%. This prevalence varies widely, and is particularly high among the most underprivileged population groups.

The status of reproductive health among young people is indicated by levels of unintended pregnancies and sexually transmitted diseases (STDs). For those Member States for which complete data are available, teenage abortion rates per 1,000 women range from 5 to 22 (8 to 28 in the age group 20-24); these rates are basically at the same level as they were in the mid-80s. Chlamydia is by far the most common of the sexually transmitted diseases, carried by 5-7 % of young people. Very little is known about the true incidence of HIV infections among 15-24-year-old people. From 1992 to 1997 the annual number of new cases of AIDS in the age group 15-24 decreased from about 1,050 cases to about 460.

In the field of lifestyles, the following findings are particularly noteworthy:

■ Experiments with smoking often start in childhood: 50-80 % of children aged 15 have tried smoking. In 1998, about one-fifth of all 15-year-olds were daily cigarette smokers. Regular smoking increases with age up to ages 18-20. Because of the addictive properties of nicotine, most young daily smokers continue to smoke regularly into middle age.

■ Regular alcohol consumption begins at a younger age than it used to. Although the gender gap has narrowed in many Member States, boys still drink more frequently and heavily than girls. Drinking to inebriation has become increasingly common among young people in all Member States for which comparable data are available.

■ Experimental substance abuse is common in early adolescence, but only a minority will eventually develop addictive patterns of use. Substance misuse and dependence at the age of 15-24 years is often associated with mental disorders such as depression. In the 1990s, no uniform trends in the number of deaths related to substance abuse were reported across the European Union. In the mid-1990s, among 15-16-year-olds the prevalence of experiments with cannabis ranged from 4 to 41% across the European Union; the corresponding figures for amphetamines were 1 to 13%, for cocaine 0 to 4%, for heroin 0 to 2%, for Ecstasy 0 to 9%, and for solvents 2 to 20%.

■ Although reliable data on trends in physical activity are not available, there is evidence that many young people are not participating in sufficient levels of physical activity to attain health benefits. The rising trend in obesity is particularly alarming.

The following areas are considered priority issues for future activity:

■ There is a clear need to improve the quality and comparability of data, to develop comparative indicators of health and to analyse both the statistical information and the research findings in the differing contexts of the individual Member States. New comparative studies on the health and well-being of young people should also cover mental, social and cultural aspects, and try to explain differences between countries by relating them to structural and/or cultural factors; they could thus play an important part in the further development of comprehensive reporting on young people's health in the EU.

■ The major challenges with respect to improving young people's health in the EU are linked to the social and regional inequalities in health that are caused by economic, social and cultural determinants of ill-health.

■ Attention should be paid not only to health-related lifestyles (smoking, abuse of alcohol and other substances, nutrition, physical activity), but also to the mental health of young people. Moreover, premature deaths from accidents and suicides call for urgent preventive action.

■ The above information is the executive summary of *The state of young people's health in the European Union*, produced by the European Commission.

© European Commission

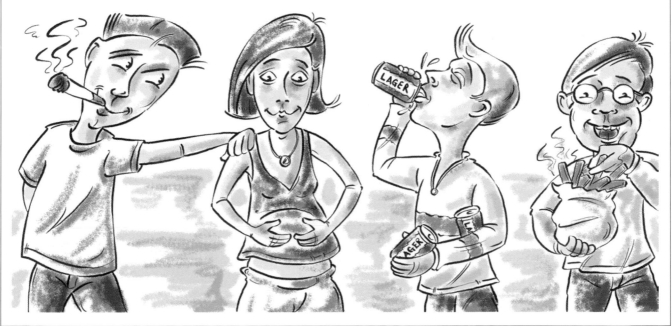

Teenage sex shock

One youngster in every 14 has sex in their first teenage year

One youngster in every 14 has sex in their first teenage year, research has revealed.

But many deeply regret it, and say they wish they had waited.

Among girls, 36 per cent were 'unhappy' over losing their virginity at 13, and 18 per cent said 'it should never have happened'.

Even among boys, some 32 per cent admitted they regretted having early sex.

Many youngsters had intercourse while under the influence of drink or drugs, according to the report by the Institute of Education and University College London.

The findings reinforce evidence that the legal age of consent – 16 – is being ignored by a growing number of teenagers.

But the survey results contradicted the idea that many youngsters are ignorant about contraception and need to be taught the dangers of unprotected sex.

It found that four out of five 13-year-olds who have sex do use contraception.

The research was carried out among nearly 9,000 pupils with an average age of 13 years and seven months at 27 comprehensive schools in southern England, representing a cross-section of social backgrounds.

It was part of the 'randomised trial of peer-led sex education in schools in England' – a long-running study financed by the Medical Research Council.

The survey uncovered a 'deep pool of unhappiness' among teenagers at the effect on their lives of early sex.

It found that seven per cent of 13-year-olds said they had had sex and 80 per cent had used contraception the first time.

The report added: 'There was no association between regret and

By Steve Doughty

being drunk or high (on drugs) at first sex. Reported sex was associated with lower social class, low self-esteem, dislike of school and truancy.

'More than half (53 per cent) of young people who reported having had sex had been drunk at least once a month, used drugs and smoked cigarettes.'

Youngsters who drank or used drugs, but had not had sex, were the most likely to say they were prepared to do so. Reported use of contraception at first sex was high in this age group, said researchers.

The report follows government studies suggesting high numbers of 13- and 14-year-olds are now sexually active.

One in four girls is reported to have had sex before the age of 16 and one in 12 has asked for contraception at a sex clinic at the age of 14.

Sex education in schools and

government initiatives to reduce teenage pregnancies have concentrated recently on condoning sexual behaviour but encouraging teenagers to use contraceptives.

However, researcher Vicki Strange pointed out that the findings of the latest survey showed that contraceptive use among 13-year-olds was already widespread.

The findings brought fresh criticism by family groups of the Government's attitude to sex and teenagers.

Robert Whelan, of Family and Youth Concern, said: 'Ministers base their strategy on the idea that young people have a right to a sex life just like adults.

'But a high proportion of teenagers were not in a position to make a valid choice because they were drunk or drugged – and a high number deeply regretted it afterwards.'

He added: 'These children are too young to cope with sexual relationships, and that's why there is an age of consent of 16.'

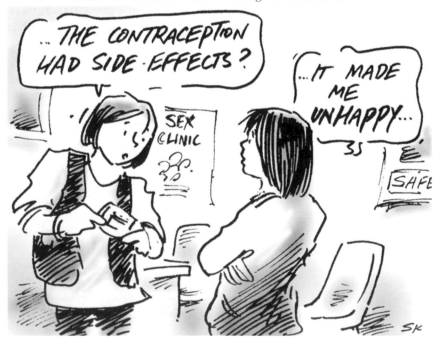

Alarm over new 'superbug'

Doctors are battling against a new strain of a sexually transmitted disease that can rob women of their fertility.

Standard antibiotics are failing to cure an alarming one in ten cases of gonorrhoea. Now a surge in the number of sufferers is thought to have led to the rise of a gonorrhoea 'superbug'.

Overuse of antibiotics encourages bacteria to mutate and become resistant, which renders the drugs powerless.

Four out of five 13-year-olds who have sex do use contraception

---

Experts blame increasing promiscuity, particularly among the young, for the rise in cases of gonorrhoea.

It can lead to pelvic inflammatory disease in women and mean they may suffer blocked fallopian tubes.

After chlamydia, it is the UK's most common bacterial sexual infection.

Cases have risen by 87 per cent in women and men since 1996 to 22,697.

The biggest surge has taken place among 16- to 19-year-olds, where cases soared by 122 per cent between 2001 and 1996.

© The Daily Mail
April, 2003

Teenage pregnancy and parenthood

Information from the Health Development Agency

Introduction

It is widely understood that teenage pregnancy and early motherhood can be associated with poor educational achievement, poor physical and mental health, social isolation, poverty and related factors. There is also a growing recognition that socio-economic disadvantage can be both a cause and a consequence of teenage parenthood.

Teenage pregnancy and parenthood in the UK

The UK has the highest rate of teenage pregnancies in western Europe (UNICEF, 2001). Throughout most of the region, birth rates to teenage mothers fell during the 1970s, but UK rates have been fairly consistent, staying relatively stable since 1969 (Botting et al., 1998). Between 1998 and 2000, the under-18 and under-16 conception rates have fallen by over 6%, and:
- In 2000, 38,690 under- 18-year-olds in England became pregnant
- 44.8% of these ended in legal abortion
- 7,617 of these conceptions were to under-16s
- 54.5% of conceptions to under-16s ended in legal abortion (Office for National Statistics, 2000).

In 1998, the Social Exclusion Unit (SEU) was asked by the Prime Minister to study the causes of teenage pregnancy and to develop a strategy to reduce the high rates of teenage pregnancy and parenthood in England. The SEU published its report, *Teenage Pregnancy* (SEU, 1999), and this provides a comprehensive review of the area and identifies the most effective approaches to tackle teenage pregnancy.

The main aims of the national strategy are to:
- Reduce the rate of teenage conceptions, with the specific aim

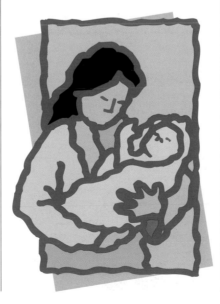

of halving the rate of conceptions among under- 18-year-olds by 2010. *The NHS Plan* provides a target for an interim reduction of 15% by 2004
- Set a firmly established downward trend in the under-16 conception rates by 2010
- Reduce inequality in rates between the 20% of wards with the highest rate of teenage conception and the average wards by at least 25%
- Increase to 60% the participation of teenage parents in education, training and employment to reduce their risk of long-term social exclusion by 2010.

That report sets out a ten-year national strategy for meeting these aims, and a concerted programme of national and regional work, co-ordinated by the cross-government Teenage Pregnancy Unit (TPU), is under way.

Who becomes a teenage parent?

Girls and young women from social class V are at approximately ten times the risk of becoming teenage mothers as girls and young women from social class I. Young people with below-average achievement levels at ages 7 and 16 have also been found to be at significantly higher risk of becoming teenage parents (Kiernan, 1995).

We know less about who becomes a young father (but the above refers to young parents). Evidence suggests (Kiernan, 1995) that young fathers (defined as those who became fathers before the age of 22), like young mothers, are more likely to come from lower socio-economic groups, from families that have experienced financial difficulties, and are more likely than average to have left school at the minimum age.

There is some evidence that certain groups of young people seem to be particularly vulnerable to becoming teenage parents. They include:

- Young people in or leaving care (Biehal, 1995)
- Homeless young people (JRF, 1995)
- School excludees, truants and young people under-performing at school (Kiernan, 1995)
- Children of teenage mothers (Botting et al., 1998)
- Members of some ethnic minority groups (Botting et al., 1998; Berthoud, 2001) – for example, Caribbean, Pakistani and Bangladeshi women are more likely than white women to have been teenage mothers
- Young people involved in crime (Botting et al., 1998)
- Conception rates are slightly higher in the north of England than the south, although there is a lot of regional variation (Botting et al., 1998).

What happens to teenage parents and their children?

Although parenthood can be a positive and life-enhancing experience for some young people, it may also bring a number of negative consequences for young parents and their children. These factors include:

- Negative short-, medium- and long-term health and mental health outcomes for young mothers (Botting et al., 1998)
- Education and employment – as well as being more likely to have problems at school before they become pregnant, young mothers are less likely to complete their

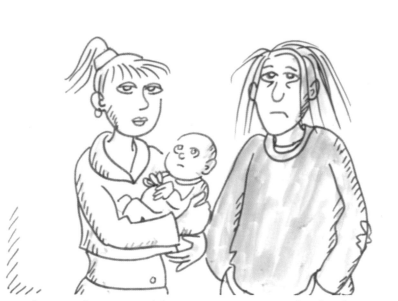

education, have no qualifications by age 33, be in receipt of benefits and if employed be on lower incomes than their peers (SEU, 1999)

- Housing – 80% of under-18 mothers live in someone else's household (e.g. parents) (Botting et al., 1998), and teenagers are more likely to have to move house during pregnancy
- Family – teenage mothers are more likely to be lone parents (Kiernan, 1995), and more likely to find themselves in the middle of family conflict (SEU, 1999)
- Young fathers – although there is little data on this group, health, economic and employment outcomes for young fathers post-parenthood seem to be similar to those of young mothers (Kiernan, 1995).

There may also be negative outcomes for the babies and children of teenage mothers:

- Babies tend to have a lower than average birth weight (Botting et al., 1998)
- Infant mortality in this group is 60% higher than for babies of older women (Berthoud, 2001)
- Some 44% of mothers under 20 breastfeed, compared to 64% of 20- 24-year-olds and up to 80% of older mothers (Botting et al., 1998)
- Children of teenage mothers are more likely to have the experience of being a lone-parent family, and are generally at

increased risk of poverty, poor housing and having bad nutrition (Botting et al., 1998)

- Daughters of teenage mothers may be more likely to become teenage parents themselves (Botting et al., 1998; Kiernan, 1995).

■ This briefing presents the current evidence from selected systematic and other reviews and meta-analyses published since 1996. The full review – Swann, C., Bowe, K., McCormick, G., Kosmin, M. (2003) *Teenage pregnancy and parenthood: a review of reviews*. London: HDA – will be updated regularly as new evidence becomes available. It can be accessed via: www.hda-online.org.uk/ evidence It seeks to pull together learning from review-level data about effective interventions to reduce the rates of teenage pregnancy and improve the outcomes for teenage parents.

Authors of this review:
C. Swann, K. Bowe, G. McCormick & M. Kosmin
Acknowledgements:
Dr Catherine Dennison; Dr Roger Ingham; Rachel Thomson; Suzanne Speak; Lynda Clark; Kaye Wellings

■ The above information is from the Health Development Agency's web site which can be found at www.hda-online.org.uk

Teenage sexual activity

Statistics and trends

First sexual experience
The age at which young people today report their first experience of sex is 14 for women and 13 for men.[1]

First sexual intercourse
The age at which the majority of 16-19-year-olds today first have sexual intercourse is 16. Almost 30% of young men and almost 26% of young women report having intercourse before their 16th birthday. By the age of 20 the vast majority of young people today have had sexual intercourse.[2]

Homosexual experience
Among 16- 24-year-olds, 5% of men and 2% of women report some homosexual experience with 7% and 5% respectively saying they have experienced homosexual attraction.[2]

Trends in sexual behaviour
There has been a sharp drop in the age at first intercourse over the last 50 years. Twenty-six per cent of young women today experience sexual intercourse before the age of 16 compared with fewer than 1% of those who were young in the 1950s. Among young men, 30% report intercourse before 16 compared with 6% of men in the 1950s. The age at first sexual experience has also dropped years from 16 to 14 for women and from 15 to 13 for men. However, the time between first experience and first intercourse is shortening, particularly for women. Young women today now have intercourse about 2 years after their first sexual experience compared with 4 years during the 1950s.[2]

Is the pill responsible for young people having sex earlier?
The biggest drop in age at first intercourse, from 21 to 19, occurred during the 1950s. The age of first intercourse fell as much during this one decade as it did over the next 30 years. This was before the introduction of the pill in 1961, which did not become widely available to unmarried women until 1972.[1]

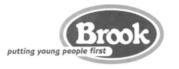

Reasons for first intercourse
Young people cite natural follow-on, being in love and curiosity as the main reasons why they had first intercourse. Although young men are more likely to say they had intercourse out of curiosity and women because they are in love, there has been a steady convergence between the sexes on the reasons for first intercourse.[1]

Peer pressure
Although the majority of young people do not report having first intercourse because of peer pressure, young men are twice as likely as women to cite pressure from peers as the main reason for losing their virginity. Among teenage women claiming they were pressurised into first intercourse, 82% said the pressure came from boyfriends.[1]

Feelings about first intercourse
Among 16- 24-year-olds, 20% of men and 42% of women felt they had intercourse too soon. The younger the age at first intercourse, the more likely the regret.[2]

Factors associated with first intercourse under 16

Early sexual experience
The earlier the age of first sexual experience, the younger the age at first intercourse.

Early menarche
Women who first menstruate at 13 or older are much less likely to have sex under 16 than those who start their periods under 13.[2]

Educational achievements
Median age at first intercourse increases with educational level. Young people reaching at least GCSE standard education are less likely to have intercourse before the age of 16.

Sex education
Young people who cite friends and the media as their main sources of information about sex have first sexual intercourse younger than those who report school sex education as their main source.

Patterns of sexual relationships
The majority of young people have their first sexual intercourse in an established relationship but intercourse under 16 is more likely to take place with a new partner.

Young people are increasingly likely to plan their first sexual intercourse. As planned intercourse is more likely to be protected, this trend is likely to increase contraceptive use among teenagers.

Fewer than 1% of young people are married at the time of first sexual intercourse. Serial monogamy is still the most common pattern of sexual relationships among young people.

The percentage of young men having their first sexual intercourse with a prostitute has steadily declined over the last 40 years. This was reported by 3.4% of men who were young in the 1950s compared with 0% of young men today.[3]

International comparisons
The age at which young people today report having first sexual intercourse does not vary significantly between developed countries.

References
1   K Wellings et al, *Sexual Behaviour in Britain*, Penguin 1994.
2   K Wellings et al, Sexual behaviour in Britain: early heterosexual experience, *The Lancet*, Vol 358, December 1 2001
3   A. Johnson et al. *Sexual behaviour in Britain: partnerships and high risk behaviours*. The Lancet, Vol. 358, December 2001.

■ The above information is from a factsheet from Brook's web site which can be found at www.brook.org.uk

© Brook Advisory Centres

Drug use among young people

Prevalence of taking drugs

In 2001, 29% of pupils reported that they had ever tried one or more drugs, 20% had taken drugs in the last year and 12% had done so in the last month. Boys were slightly more likely than girls to have taken drugs – among boys 13% had taken drugs in the last month and 21% had taken drugs in the last year, compared with 11% and 19% respectively among girls.

As pupils get older, they become much more likely to take drugs: only 3% of 11-year-olds and 4% of 12-year olds had taken drugs in the last month, but 24% of 15-year-olds had. Almost half (48%) of 15-year-olds had ever tried drugs at some point and 29% had taken drugs in the last year.

It is not possible to compare these figures from 2001 with the results from previous surveys in the series due to changes in the structure and wording of questions. However, responses to other questions (such as drug use among friends and attitudes towards experimentation with drugs) suggest that the increase in drug taking reported between 1998 and 2000 has probably continued into 2001. A full methodological explanation is detailed in the main report.

Proportions who had taken cannabis and Class A drugs in last year

Cannabis was by far the most widely taken drug. Thirteen per cent of pupils reported taking this drug in the last year. Seven per cent had sniffed volatile substances. Every other individual drug had been taken in the last year by no more than 3% of pupils, with a total of 4% taking any Class A drug in the last year. At age 15, four in ten had taken at least one drug in the last twelve months, most of whom had taken cannabis. Nine per cent had taken at least one Class A drug, though cocaine and

heroin had respectively been taken in the last year by only 3% and 1% of 15-year-olds.

Prevalence of sniffing volatile substances

Reported levels of misuse of volatile substances (sniffing or inhaling glue, gas, aerosols or other solvents) were much higher than in previous surveys in the series, although this is almost certainly due to the change in question format rather than a sudden change in the actual levels of misuse.

The patterns of prevalence of misuse of volatile substances were different to those seen for other behaviours. Older pupils were more likely than younger pupils to smoke, drink or take cannabis, but misuse of volatile substances did not show a strong relationship with age. Use of volatile substances in the last year was highest among 13- and 14-year-olds at 9% and lowest among 11-year-olds at 4%.

It is possible to distinguish between first-time users of a drug in the last year and 'repeat' users by comparing the age at which pupils first took a drug with their current age. Despite the relatively high

prevalence of pupils who had ever sniffed volatile substances, repeat usage was low – the proportion of pupils who were classified as repeat users of volatile substances was 4% or less for each age group. In contrast repeat use of cannabis increased with age – less than 1% of 11-year-olds were repeat users of cannabis, but this had increased to 16% of 15-year-olds.

Type of drugs taken at age when first took drugs

For each drug, pupils who had ever tried it were asked at what age they first tried it. From this it is possible to work out at what age pupils first tried drugs and which drugs were taken by them at this age.

Pupils tended to have only tried one drug at the age when they first tried drugs, with 45% reporting that they had only sniffed volatile substances and 41% reporting that they had only tried cannabis at the age when they had first tried drugs. The similarity in the overall percentages having tried only volatile substances or only cannabis masks a very strong relationship with the age at which drugs were first tried. Eighty-

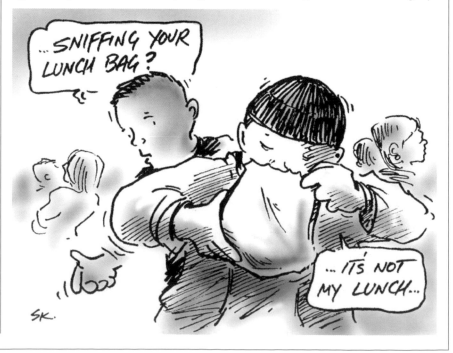

SK.

six per cent of pupils whose first use of drugs was at age 10 or younger took volatile substances and no other drugs at that age compared with 7% who took only cannabis. In contrast, among pupils whose first use of drugs was at age 15, 74% took cannabis and no other drugs at that age compared with 8% who took only volatile substances.

Relationships between volatile substances, cannabis, smoking, drinking and Class A drugs

There was a stronger link between taking cannabis and smoking and drinking than there was between taking volatile substances and smoking and drinking. Around half of those who had taken cannabis in the last year were regular smokers and half usually drank at least twice a week, whereas among those who had taken volatile substances in the last year the equivalent proportions were both around a third.

It is possible to determine whether taking volatile substances, cannabis or smoking or drinking are risk factors for later use of Class A drugs by restricting analysis to pupils who are currently aged 15, and had not taken Class A drugs by age 13. By looking at this group, it is possible to see which behaviours at 13 were most likely to predict whether pupils had taken Class A drugs by 15. Fifteen-year-old pupils who had taken cannabis by the age of 13 were the most likely to have taken Class A drugs in the last year (31% compared with 5% of those who had not taken cannabis by this age).

There was a weaker link between taking volatile substances and future use of Class A drugs – those who had taken volatile substances by age 13 were more likely than those who had not to have taken Class A drugs in the last year (16% compared with 7% respectively).

These results suggest that taking cannabis is more likely to lead to future use of Class A drugs than not taking cannabis. However, this does not imply that pupils necessarily progress from taking cannabis to taking Class A drugs; 69% of those who had taken cannabis by age 13 had not taken Class A drugs in the last year.

Awareness of drugs

There was widespread awareness of illegal drugs among young people in

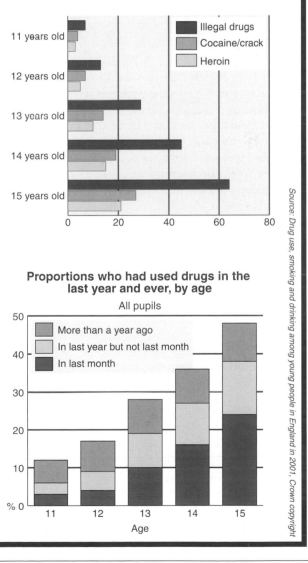

Young people and drugs

Reasons for taking drugs on first and last occasion

All ever taken drugs/All taken drugs in last month
(except those who had only taken volatile substances)

- See what it was like
- Get high/feel good
- Friends doing it
- Nothing better to do
- Forget problems
- Offered drugs
- Dare
- Cool

First occasion
Last occasion

0 10 20 30 40 50 60 70%

Proportion perceiving it would be easy to obtain drugs

All pupils

- 11 years old
- 12 years old
- 13 years old
- 14 years old
- 15 years old

Illegal drugs
Cocaine/crack
Heroin

0 20 40 60 80

Awareness of different types of drugs

All pupils

- Cocaine
- Heroin
- Cannabis
- Crack
- Ecstasy
- Tranquillisers
- Magic mushrooms
- LSD
- Amphetamines
- Anabolic steroids
- Methadone
- Poppers

0 20 40 60 80 100%

Proportions who had used drugs in the last year and ever, by age

All pupils

- More than a year ago
- In last year but not last month
- In last month

50
40
30
20
10
% 0

11 12 13 14 15
Age

Source: Drug use, smoking and drinking among young people in England in 2001, Crown copyright

England. In 2001, 94% of pupils had heard of cocaine, 93% of cannabis and 91% of heroin. At least eight out of ten pupils had heard of crack (84%) and ecstasy (81%), and at least seven out of ten pupils had heard of tranquillisers (74%) and magic mushrooms (74%). Even the less well-known drugs recorded awareness levels over 50% – LSD (64%), amphetamines (57%), anabolic steroids (55%), methadone (55%) and poppers (52%). Only 2% had never heard of any of the drugs listed.

Awareness of every type of drug increased with age. Yet even at age 11 there was high awareness of cocaine (84%), heroin (81%) and cannabis (75%), though limited awareness of amphetamines (19%), poppers (24%) and LSD (27%). By age 15 virtually all pupils had heard of cocaine, heroin, cannabis, crack and ecstasy. Even the least well-known drug, methadone, was recognised by 69%.

Knowledge of drugs

Pupils' knowledge of the potential physical effects of drugs was assessed through a series of 7 statements, four true and three false. Summing the number of statements which pupils answered correctly illustrates the extent to which knowledge of drugs increased with age. At age 11, 15% of pupils gave five or more correct answers out of a possible seven. This proportion then climbs steadily to reach 54% among 15-year-olds, a level which implies a good deal of basic knowledge among older pupils but also a substantial degree of remaining ignorance.

Pupils' knowledge of drugs was related to their use of cannabis, but not to their use of Class A drugs. Among 15-year-old pupils, use of cannabis in the last month was higher among pupils who got five or more answers correct (23%) than among those who got a maximum of two answers correct (17%).

■ The above information is from *Drug use, smoking and drinking among young people in England in 2001*. A survey carried out on behalf of the Department of Health by the National Centre for Social Research and the National Foundation for Education Research. Edited by Richard Boreham and Andrew Shaw.

© Crown copyright 2002

One in three teens 'has smoked cannabis'

Alarming levels of drug-taking, drinking and smoking among children as young as 11 have emerged in a Government survey of schools.

One in three 15-year-olds admitted trying cannabis, despite scientific studies proving that teenage users dramatically increase their risk of mental illness.

One in ten pupils regularly smokes cigarettes, leaving them at risk of lung cancer, while almost a quarter said they had drunk alcohol in the week before the poll. These pupils said they had consumed an average of 10.5 units of alcohol – the equivalent of five pints of beer, ten shots of spirits or ten glasses of wine.

Levels of alcohol abuse by children have almost doubled over the past ten years, the figures published yesterday by the Department of Health revealed.

The findings, from a survey of 10,000 pupils by the National Centre for Social Research and the National Centre for Educational Research, sparked fears that an entire generation is at risk.

By Beezy Marsh

Tory health spokesman Dr Liam Fox said: 'These are absolutely shocking social trends and in the long run it will result in a tidal wave of ill-health which will threaten to swamp the health service.'

Overall, 18 per cent of pupils aged 11 to 15 said they had taken drugs in the previous 12 months.

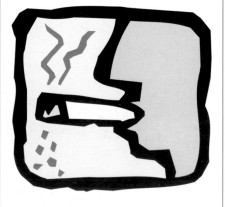

Cannabis was the narcotic of choice, with 13 per cent having tried it in the past year. By the age of 15, that number had risen to 31 per cent.

A total of 28 per cent of pupils said they have been offered cannabis. Researchers have recently discovered that those who started using cannabis in their teens were four times more likely to be diagnosed with a psychiatric disorder.

Ministers have been accused of sending out messages that the drug is virtually risk-free by downgrading it legally. The decision, which comes into force this summer, will end police powers to arrest people caught smoking cannabis.

Harder drugs, including cocaine, ecstasy and amphetamines, have been touted to one in five school children, the schools study showed.

A Department of Health spokesman said the number of pupils taking drugs had decreased slightly from 20 per cent in 2001 to 18 per cent in 2002.

© The Daily Mail

Models 'drive girls to smoke'

Evidence suggests more teenage girls are taking up smoking just to keep their weight down

By Beezy Marsh

More teenage girls are taking up smoking just to keep their weight down, evidence suggests.

Health experts fear they are using tobacco as an appetite suppressant, possibly influenced by images of superthin celebrities with cigarettes.

Despite advocating yoga to keep her slim, singer Geri Halliwell has been pictured smoking, as has supermodel Kate Moss.

About 26 per cent of girls aged 15 are regular smokers, compared to 21 per cent of boys of that age.

A study published in the medical journal *Tobacco Control* reveals that girls who are not bothered about their weight are less likely to take up the habit.

Researchers from Okayama University in Japan studied 273 girls aged 12 to 15 from Massachusetts, who had only tried smoking once.

They were asked to rate the value they put on being thin, using a score of 0 to 10, where 0 is 'not at all important' and 10 is 'extremely important'.

Then they were surveyed again four years later.

Almost one in four had become an established smoker, meaning they had smoked 100 or more cigarettes.

A correlation was found with those who placed a high value on being thin.

Of those who eventually progressed to smoking, just 7 per cent considered being thin to be unimportant.

> *'If a girl believes that smoking promotes weight loss she is likely to develop smoking behaviour'*

Those rating thinness as moderately important made up almost one in four of the smokers, while those who considered it extremely important accounted for almost 30 per cent.

The researchers concluded that those who considered being thin to be moderately important were more than three times as likely to smoke, while those who considered it very important were more than four times as likely.

Author Dr Kaori Honjo said: 'This is the first study to examine whether the importance of being thin is an initiating factor for smoking among younger female adolescents.

'One possibility is if a girl believes that smoking promotes weight loss she is likely to develop smoking behaviour.

'It has been unclear whether teenage girls initiate smoking with the intention to control weight, or whether dieting and smoking are part of a larger constellation of unhealthy behaviours.'

He said anti-smoking drives should include messages about healthy eating and diet to target teenage girls who may be tempted to try cigarettes to stay slim.

'This study suggests it is crucial to broaden the scope of health programmes and policies to protect adolescent health.'

© *The Daily Mail*

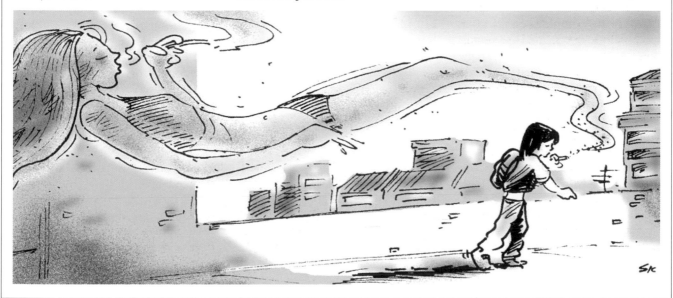

Young people and smoking

Smoking prevalence

Children become aware of cigarettes at an early age. Three out of four children are aware of cigarettes before they reach the age of 5 whether the parents smoke or not. By the age of 11 one-third of children, and by 16 years two-thirds of children have experimented with smoking. In Great Britain about 450 children start smoking every day. Large regional studies of children's smoking habits during the 1960s and 1970s showed that more boys smoked than girls and that boys started earlier. In 1982, at ASH's instigation, the government commissioned the first national survey of smoking among children and found that 11% of 11-16-year-olds were smoking regularly.

During the early nineties prevalence remained stable at 10%, but by the mid nineties teenage smoking rates were on the increase, particularly among girls. Between 1996 and 1999, there was a decline in 11- to 15-year-olds smoking regularly. The reduction in smoking prevalence occurred mainly among 14- to 15-year-olds. In 1998, the government set a target to reduce the prevalence of regular smoking among young people aged 11-15 from a baseline of 13% in 1996 to 11% by 2005 and 9% or less by 2010. Results from the 2002 survey show that prevalence of smoking has been stable since 1998. As in previous years, girls are more likely to be regular smokers than boys. The proportion of regular smokers increases sharply with age: 1% of 11-year-olds smoke regularly compared with 22% of 15-year-olds.

What factors influence children to start smoking?

Children are three times as likely to smoke if both of their parents smoke and parents' approval or disapproval of the habit is also a significant factor. Numerous studies have shown that most young smokers are influenced

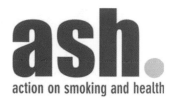

by their friends' and older siblings' smoking habits. Surveys show that children tend to smoke the brands that are promoted most heavily and advertising reinforces the smoking habit. One study of secondary school children found that a minority of smokers (38%), but a majority of non-smokers (56%), thought that tobacco advertising had quite a lot, or a lot of effect on influencing young people to start smoking. Advertising also creates the impression that smoking is a socially acceptable norm. Sports sponsorship by tobacco companies and particularly the televising of sponsored events increases children's awareness of the brands. A survey in 1996 found that around two-thirds of 11- to 16-year-

olds could identify at least one sport connected to cigarette advertising through sponsorship. Another study found that boys whose favourite sport was motor racing were twice as likely to become regular smokers than those who did not have an interest in the sport.

Smoking and children's health

Children who smoke are two to six times more susceptible to coughs and increased phlegm, wheeziness and shortness of breath than those who do not smoke. One study revealed that children who smoke are three times more likely to have time off school. The earlier children become regular smokers and persist in the habit as adults, the greater the risk of dying prematurely. A recent US study found that smoking during the teenage years causes permanent genetic changes in the lungs and forever increases the risk of lung cancer, even if the smoker subsequently stops.

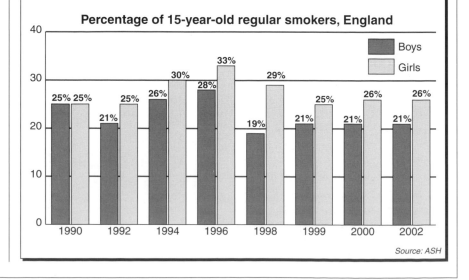

Smoking

Percentage of regular smokers aged 11-15 by sex								
Year	1990	1992	1994	1996	1998	1999	2000	2002
Boys	9	9	10	11	9	8	9	9
Girls	11	10	13	15	12	10	12	11
Total	10	10	12	13	11	9	10	10

Percentage of 15-year-old regular smokers, England

Source: ASH

Children are also more susceptible to the effects of passive smoking and nicotine levels found in the saliva of children whose parents smoke indicate that in households where both parents smoke, the children are receiving a nicotine equivalent of smoking 80 cigarettes a year. Bronchitis, pneumonia, asthma and other chronic respiratory illnesses are significantly more common in infants and children who have one or two smoking parents. Children of parents who smoke during the child's early life run a higher risk of cancer in adulthood and the larger the number of smokers in a household, the greater the cancer risk to non-smokers in the family. For a more detailed overview of the health impacts of passive smoking on children see the ASH briefing: 'Passive smoking: the impact on children'.

Addiction

Children who experiment with cigarettes quickly become addicted to the nicotine in tobacco. A MORI survey of children aged 11 to 16 years found that teenagers have similar levels of nicotine dependence as adults, with one-third of those who smoke one or more cigarettes a week lighting up their first cigarette within 30 minutes of waking up and one in twelve lighting up within the first five minutes. Over half (58%) of regular smokers aged between 11 and 15 years say that they would find it difficult to go without smoking for a week while 72% thought they would find it difficult to give up altogether. During periods of abstinence, young people experience withdrawal symptoms similar to the kind experienced by adult smokers.

Smoking prevention

Since the 1970s, health education including information about the health effects of smoking, has been included in the curriculum of most primary and secondary schools in Great Britain. Research suggests that knowledge about smoking is a necessary component of anti-smoking campaigns but by itself does not affect smoking rates. It may, however, result in a postponement of initiation. Every year, between 80,000 and 100,000 children become

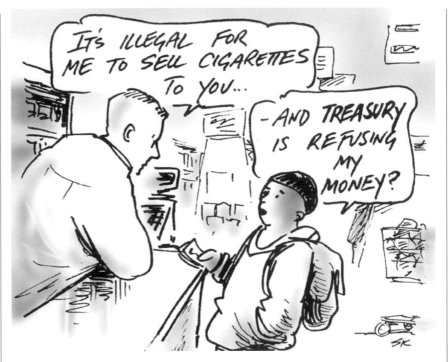

addicted to tobacco worldwide. High prices can deter children from smoking, since they do not possess a large disposable income. In Canada, when cigarette prices were raised dramatically in the 1980s and the early 1990s youth consumption of tobacco plummeted by 60%. A recent American study has shown that while price does not appear to affect initial experimentation of smoking, it is an important tool in reducing youth smoking once the habit has become established.

Children, smoking and the law

Since 1908, and currently under the Children and Young Persons (Protection from Tobacco) Act 1991, it has been illegal to sell any tobacco product to anyone below the age of 16. The Act increased the maximum fines for retailers found guilty of selling cigarettes to children to £2,500 and tightened up the previous legislation in a number of other ways.

In spite of the law, a study in 1996 revealed that the treasury received £108 million pounds in taxation from the illegal sale of cigarettes to children

---

In spite of the law, however, a study in 1996 revealed that the treasury received £108 million pounds in taxation from the illegal sale of cigarettes to children. In 1997 it was estimated that the UK tobacco industry made an annual profit of £35 million from teenage smokers.

During 2001 there were 130 prosecutions in England and Wales for underage tobacco sales, with 82 defendants being convicted and fined. Of these, 23 fines were for sums over £350. A 1998 survey found that 22% of 11- to 15-year-olds in England had tried to buy cigarettes in a shop during the previous year. Of these only 43% had been refused on at least one occasion. Legislation alone is not sufficient to prevent tobacco sales to minors. Both enforcement and community policies may improve compliance by retailers, but the impact on underage smoking prevalence using these approaches alone may still be small. Successful efforts to limit underage access to tobacco require a combination of approaches that tackle the problem comprehensively.

■ The above information is an extract from a factsheet produced by ASH, for the full text including references please visit their web site at www.ash.org.uk/html/factsheets/html/fact03.html Alternatively see page 41 for their address details.
© ASH

Conspicuous consumption

Our culture regards getting drunk as a prerequisite to having a good time – a tradition many young people are keen to continue, despite the risks

By Sarah Wellard

If you're out in any town centre on a Friday or Saturday night, you'll observe one of our great British institutions – going out with your mates and getting drunk. From recent media focus you might think this is a wholly new phenomenon, but binge drinking is nothing new and is by no means unique to Britain. As Martin Plant, professor of addiction studies and director of the Alcohol and Health Research Trust, University of the West of England, points out: 'Basically what's happening is that young people are learning from an earlier age to drink in a way that's part of our British culture. It's a north west European thing – we're in there with the Danes, Norwegians and Finns.'

> *Alcohol Concern is alarmed by the increase in alcohol consumption among children and teenagers, and especially binge drinking*

Plant believes the increase in binge drinking among young people is partly a knock-on effect of the surge in alcohol consumption that occurred after the second world war. More young people now have parents who are themselves heavy drinkers, and parents who drink heavily or abstain completely are more likely to have heavy-drinking children than are people who drink in moderation.

Disposable income is also a factor. Plant says: 'What's new is the increased spending power among 15-year-olds. It's not uncommon for them to have £30 to £50 a week pocket money.' But it's not just kids with plenty of money to spend who are drinking more. Alcohol is cheap. A pair of teenagers with only a fiver between them can get out of their heads on cider or lager from the corner shop.

Alcohol Concern is alarmed by the increase in alcohol consumption among children and teenagers, and especially binge drinking. Development officer Nicola Sinclair points out that that there are no recommended limits for children and says we know little about the effects of alcohol on bodies which are still developing. What we do know gives cause for concern – for example, children go into coma at lower blood alcohol levels than adults. Young people who have been drinking are more likely to have an accident, get into a fight or have unprotected sex. New research from Northern Ireland shows that a quarter of 15- and 16-year-olds in the province have been in trouble with the police after drinking.

Sinclair says: 'It's not just that children's bodies are less able to deal with alcohol but that they face dangers when they drink large amounts away from adult supervision, in parks or by roads or rivers. Their inexperience makes them less able to deal with the effects of alcohol and they are likely to get into trouble. They may not be prepared for the way alcohol will affect their judgement, leading for example to risky sexual behaviour.'

> *Young people who have been drinking are more likely to have an accident, get into a fight or have unprotected sex*

Pam Vedhara, youth inclusion programme (Yip) manager in South Tyneside, says it is naïve to think there is any simple solution. Levels of alcohol consumption in the North East are the highest in the UK. 'Binge drinking is the biggest factor in antisocial behaviour and disorder. We see week in week out the effects of it – vandalism, fights. Every occasion from birth to death is celebrated with drink. We measure people by alcohol, "he can't hold his drink". How can you undo the basic values of the culture?'

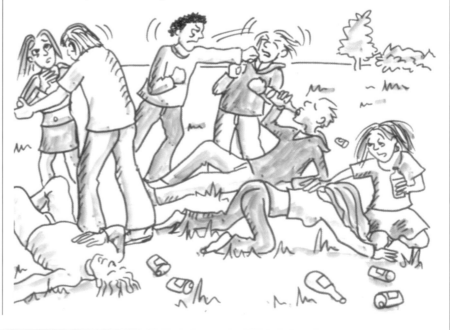

Vedhara has just launched a campaign backed by the Youth Justice Board as well as local partners to increase children's understanding of alcohol. 'The project is not initially about reducing the amount they drink,' she explains. 'It's designed to tell them what alcohol is about and sensible drinking. Most of the young people we come across, regardless of their offending behaviour, have been bombarded with stuff about lots of substances. But nobody ever tells them anything useful about drink.'

The campaign, known as Think Drink! combines awareness raising among teenagers with peer education for primary school children. Groups of 13- and 14-year-olds, including young offenders, a girls-group, Muslim young people and a group from a Roman Catholic school are

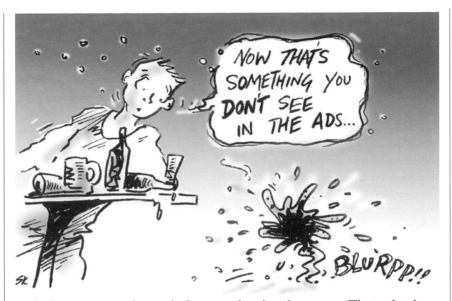

Children and alcohol

- There has been a big increase in 'binge drinking' among children and young people, with almost a third of 15- and 16-year-olds drinking more than five drinks on a single occasion in the last week – an increase of nearly 50 per cent over eight years.
- The numbers of younger children drinking alcohol has remained relatively static over the past 15 years. Some 40 per cent of 11- to 15-year-olds say they have never had a drink.
- Children and teenagers who drink are drinking more – up from 5.3 units a week in 1990 to 10.5 units in 2002.
- One in eight 11- 13-year-olds are drinking an average of nearly seven units a week – a 100 per cent increase in a decade.
- 50 per cent of 15-year-old boys drink on average the equivalent of seven pints of beer a week.
- One in seven over-16s say they have had unprotected sex after drinking.
- One in eight 15- and 16-year-olds have been injured or involved in an accident after drinking.

embarking on an eight-week Open College accredited course on issues such as alcohol and health, sex and alcohol and alcohol and the law. As part of the course they will be involved in making a video, a website and posters focusing on healthy-drinking messages. Some of the participants will then go into primary schools to talk about drinking.

Overall, research suggests that most public education is ineffective. Hardly surprising given the billions spent by the drinks industry on advertising

---

Vedhara believes that peer education is an effective way of getting young people to listen to a message, and the peer educators themselves benefit from increased self-esteem. 'If you watch a video that has been produced to near professional quality and the people who made it are the big people in your classroom, it's extremely powerful,' she says. But from experience with young people in the Yip she knows how difficult it is to change drinking behaviour. 'We try to get people to see the connection between drinking at seven-thirty and being locked up at half-past ten. It's a drip, drip, drip approach but I wouldn't pretend we've had huge

levels of success. Their drinking simply mirrors the social behaviour of the adults they see.'

According to Sinclair, there are examples of education programmes which have been effective. But overall, research suggests that most public education is ineffective. Hardly surprising given the billions spent by the drinks industry on advertising and the low priority accorded by the government to healthy-drinking messages compared say with drugs education. So far, government curbs on advertising have left alcohol alone, although this may change when the new strategy on alcohol is published later this year.

Plant believes the way forward is to focus on controls on public drinking and stricter enforcement of licensing such as penalties for serving underage customers or people who are already drunk. He says: 'At the level of individual pubs and bars there is a lot of irresponsible marketing with no concern for the consequences, like happy hours and clubs which offer young women free drinks all night. It's on the streets where a lot of the trouble happens – in the queues for buses and taxis and fast food.' He adds: 'Kids are always going to push at the limits. The ideal way is to put some controls around the places where they do drink.'

■ The above information is from *0-19 Magazine*, their web site can be found at www.zero2nineteen.co.uk

Alcohol sales to underage adolescents

Information from the Alcohol Education and Research Council

Introduction

A number of recent studies have reported high levels of alcohol consumption among adolescents in the UK. Ease of access to alcohol may be one important factor.

This study, carried out by Professor Paul Willner and his colleagues at the University of Wales, Swansea, used a variety of methods to investigate the availability of alcohol to underage drinkers. First, they asked British adolescents how easy they found it to purchase alcohol from different types of outlet as well as the extent to which sales are actually made to underage customers. A test-purchasing study was then carried out.

This involved 13- and 16-year-old adolescents attempting to purchase alcohol. They also assessed the attitudes of alcohol vendors to underage sales, vendors' ability to judge the ages of their underage customers, and the effectiveness of a police intervention intended to reduce underage alcohol purchases.

Findings

- Young people report that alcohol is freely available, from a variety of different types of outlet, to underage adolescents who wish to purchase it.
- The young people's views were corroborated by test-purchase observations confirming that 16-year-old girls and boys, and girls as young as 13, have little difficulty in buying alcohol.
- Challenging young people on their age at the point of sale may deter them to some extent from buying alcohol. However, challenges are rarely issued, and little use is being made of the 'Prove It' scheme, at least in the areas studied.
- The overwhelming majority of vendors tested were keen to sell alcohol to minors.
- Underage purchasers were still sold alcohol even after showing a card that displayed their date of birth.
- There was little difference between different types of outlet in their willingness to sell alcohol to minors. In particular, there was no support for the public perception that the problem of underage alcohol sales resides mainly in corner shops, and that the chain supermarkets have put their houses in order.
- Vendors perceive little risk in selling alcohol to minors.
- Vendors overestimate the age of underage customers, particularly girls. However, age-estimation errors were not sufficient to account for the full extent of underage alcohol sales.
- The police intervention failed to decrease sales. This suggests that vendors do not change their behaviour in response to the threat of legal action.

Implications

- Earlier onsets of drinking have been linked to increased risks of alcohol and drug problems in later life. It has also been shown repeatedly that restricting the availability of alcohol to young people decreases deaths and injuries through road traffic accidents. It follows that the easy availability of alcohol documented in the present report has significant adverse consequences for young people's mental and physical health.
- As alcohol vendors appear to overestimate the age of their underage customers, there may be some scope to reduce underage sales by vendor training programmes aimed at improving the ability of vendors to judge young people's ages accurately, and encouraging them to err on the side of caution.
- Training programmes to increase vendors' confidence to request proof of age, together with more reliable proof-of-age schemes are also recommended.

Alcohol sales

The table below shows the proportion of test-purchase attempts that resulted in sales of alcohol to 13-year-old and 16-year-old girls and boys. The lower part of each bar shows sales that were made without challenge and the upper part shows sales that were made following an age challenge.

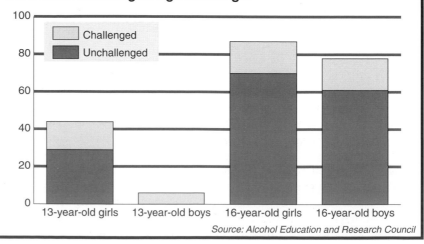

Source: Alcohol Education and Research Council

- Test-purchasing methods are used by police and trading standards officers in the enforcement of age restrictions on the sale of a variety of commodities (e.g. tobacco, fireworks and pornography). However, alcohol differs from these other commodities in that it is illegal not only for the vendor to sell alcohol but also for the underage purchaser to buy it. This legal anomaly has meant that, while several police forces use test purchasing to identify vendors who sell alcohol to children, the evidence obtained in these operations is almost never used to bring prosecutions or to remove alcohol licences. The present data suggest that a change in the law is needed to legalise test purchases of alcohol and so enable more effective enforcement of the minimum age laws. The easy availability of alcohol to young people would then be likely to decrease.

- Copies of the full report can be obtained from the AERC. There will be £10.00 handling charge for a hard copy. An electronic copy can be sent by e-mail free of charge.

- The above information is from *Alcohol Insight 1*. Alcohol Insights are brief summaries of research or action projects funded by the AERC. Visit their web site at www.aerc.org.uk
© *Alcohol Education and Research Council (AERC)*

Young people's drinking

Information from Alcohol Concern

Drinking among young people is a major issue of concern for parents and people working with young people particularly in relation to the risks of excess drinking. This article looks at research into young people's drinking. It indicates the prevalence of drinking, trends in drinking patterns and highlights alcohol-related problems that are specific to young people. The focus is on young people under sixteen.

Recent trends
While the proportion of 11-15-year-olds who don't drink at all has remained at about 40% since 1988, some disturbing trends have emerged in recent years

- Young people are drinking larger amounts of alcohol. The average amount drunk by 11-15-year-olds in 1990 was 0.8 units per week, rising to 1.6 units in 1998.[1] Amongst 11-15-year-olds who drink, average consumption rose from 5.3 units in 1990 to 10.4 units in 2000, but fell in 2001 to 9.8 units.[2,6]
- Binge drinking is common among young people in the UK, with 56% of 15-16-year-olds having drunk more than 5 drinks on a single occasion in the last 30 days. 30% of this age group report this behaviour 3 or more times in the last 30 days.[3] Comparison with an earlier edition of this survey shows that the proportion of young people who binge has increased from 22% in 1995 to 30% in 1999.
- The proportion of 11-15-year-olds who drink at least once a week has fluctuated over the last decade rising from 21% in 1990 to 27% in 1996 but dropping suddenly to 21% again in 2000. By 2001 the proportion had risen again to 26% of 11-15 year olds drinking at least once a week.[2,6]
- Young people are drinking larger amounts of alcohol. The average amount drunk by 11-15-year-olds in 1990 was 0.8 units per week, rising to 1.6 units in 1998.[1] Amongst 11-15-year-olds who drink, the average rose from 5.3 units in 1990 to 10.4 units in 2000.[2]
- There is a sharp increase in prevalence of drinking with age. In 2000 5% of all pupils aged 11 had drunk in the previous week compared to 49% of 15-year-olds.[2] Note that a recent study by the Schools Health Education Unit (2001) indicates that the proportion of students who drank at least one drink in the last week is as high as 19% of 11-year-old boys and 13% of 11-year-old girls. However, the proportion of 15-year-olds drinking the previous week is roughly similar to that in the DoH study.[4]

A comparative European study of drinking among 15-16-year-olds (ESPAD) showed that UK figures for alcohol consumption were some of the highest in Europe alongside Ireland and Denmark:
- 94% of 15- 16-year-olds have consumed alcohol at least once, with 47% having drunk alcohol at least 40 times compared to 20% of 15-16-year-olds in France and 15% of this age group in Portugal.[3]
- The UK also comes near the top of the list where consumption in the last 30 days is concerned with 16% of 15- 16-year-olds in the UK having drunk alcohol more than 10 times in the last 30 days.[3]

A recent (2002) survey of more than 14,000 students in secondary schools in England, Scotland and Wales, found that:
- Six out of 10 boys and 50% of girls aged 11-12 had tried at least one alcoholic drink.
- Of this age group 9% of boys and 5% of girls described themselves as regular drinkers. This figure rises to 39% of boys and 33% of girls amongst 15-16 year olds.
- Eight out of 10 students aged 15-16 had drunk alcohol in the previous month.
- 43% of students aged 14-15 and 50% of 15- 16-year-olds had consumed five or more alcoholic drinks in a single session – binge drinking.

- More than 25% of students aged 15-16 reported 3 or more binge drinking sessions in the past month.
- Over 60% of students reported that they had drunk alcohol before the age of 13 and 1 in 7 students said that they began drinking at least once a week.[5]

(There are a range of national and international surveys of young people's drinking behaviour employing different sampling methods and survey techniques. The majority of these surveys are based on self-reported consumption patterns but in the case DoH the authors report that the young people's responses are generally truthful. Many of the statistics in this article are drawn from large-scale surveys to provide an indication of the current situation.)

References
1 Goddard, E. and Higgins, V. *Smoking, Drinking and Drug Use among teenagers in 1998*, ONS, 1999.
2 Boreham, R. & Shaw, A. (Eds), (2001) *Smoking, drinking and drug use among young teenagers in 2000*: A survey carried out on behalf of the Department of Health by the National Centre for Social Research and the National Foundation for Educational Research, The Stationery Office, London.
3 Hibell, B. et al (2000) *The 1999 European School Survey Project on Alcohol and other Drugs* (ESPAD), CAN.
4 Balding, J. (2001) *Young people in 2000: legal and illegal drugs*, Schools Health Education Unit. Exeter.
5 Beinart, S. et al (2002) *Youth at risk? A national survey of risk factors, protective factors and problem behaviour among young people in England, Scotland and Wales*, Communities that Care, London.
6 Department of Health (2002), *Drug Use, smoking and drinking among young teenagers in 2001*: A survey carried out on behalf of the Department of Health by the National Centre for Social Research and the National Foundation for Educational Research, The Stationery Office, London.

- The above information from Alcohol Concern's web site can be found at www.alcoholconcern.org.uk
© Alcohol Concern

UK youth too busy to 'get physical'

Key findings

- 7- to 10-year-old kids tend to do less structured sporting activities but were more likely to play outside actively with their friends – less than half of these are aware that this can help them be fit and healthy.
- 11- to 13-year-olds get the most from physical activity. At this age, children are learning to be sociable, making friends and do not have the exam pressures of the older kids. This age group is the most physically active and enjoys exercise the most.
- 14- to 16-year-olds are starting to feel the pressures of exams – 56% feel that study is more important than physical activity. They are also becoming self-conscious and other interests may be becoming more important. They are less likely to 'play actively' in the same way as younger children and are the most reluctant to exercise.
- A third of all young people (33%) feel they will look better and get a better body if they are fit and healthy. Response was highest in the body-conscious teen years with 41% of 14- to 16-year-olds believing it was a key element of being fit.
- One in five 14- to 16-year-olds believed that becoming fitter and healthier meant hard work, as opposed to only 12% of 7- to 10-year-olds.

When asked how they spent their break times at school, 70% of 7- to 10-year-olds say they play actively compared with only 3% of 14- to 16-year-olds

---

- Boys are more likely than girls to do exercise because it makes them healthy (56% compared to 48%), while girls are likely to do exercise to look good and lose weight (11% compared to 4%).
- Those who do physical activities, such as sport, are far more likely to be boys (67% compared to 47% girls). Girls (33% to 23% boys) and younger children (37% 7-10s compared to 23% 11-16s) are more likely to do activities which are not sport related.
- When asked how they spent their break times at school, 70% of 7- to 10-year-olds say they play actively compared with only 3% of 14- to 16-year-olds.
- In terms of attitudes to physical activity, children from higher socio-economic groups tend to be encouraged by their parents more and see the fun and sociable side of exercise as opposed to those in lower socio-economic groups.
- 34% of young people see David Beckham as the celebrity they most think of as being really fit and healthy. Michael Owen is the second most mentioned, mostly by boys (27% to 16%). Geri Halliwell is the third most nominated, by 16% – all of which are girls.
- The above information is from MORI's web site which can be found at www.mori.com
© 2003 MORI

Diet and nutrition

A summary of the Findings of the National Diet and Nutrition Survey of young people aged 4-18

Introduction

The report is the findings of a survey of the diet and nutrition of a representative sample of 2672 young people aged 4 to 18 years. The last such survey, 'The Diets of British Schoolchildren', was conducted in 1983. The report is part of the National Diet and Nutrition Survey (NDNS) programme which examines different sectors of the population and was jointly set up by the Ministry of Agriculture, Fisheries and Food and the Department of Health in 1992. Responsibility for the NDNS programme has now been transferred to the Food Standards Agency.

Foods and drinks consumed

White bread, savoury snacks, potato chips, biscuits, boiled, mashed and jacket potatoes and chocolate confectionery were the most commonly consumed foods by young people in the survey, eaten by more than 80% of the group during the seven-day dietary record.

Breakfast cereals

About 50% ate wholegrain and high-fibre breakfast cereals, but boys were more likely than girls to eat 'other' cereals (74% vs 64%).

Meat

The most commonly consumed type of meat was chicken and turkey dishes, eaten by over 70% of young people.

Salad and vegetables

47% of boys and 59% of girls ate raw and salad vegetables (excluding tomatoes), around 40% of the group ate cooked leafy green vegetables and about 60% other cooked vegetables.

Fruit

The most commonly consumed fruits were apples and pears, eaten by over half the group, followed by bananas

By Sara Price

eaten by just under 40%. A quarter of young people ate citrus fruit and about a third ate 'other' fruit (mainly soft fruit).

Drinks

Three-quarters of young people drank standard carbonated soft drinks and 45% drank low calorie versions. Fruit juice was consumed by 46% of boys and 51% of girls. Tea was consumed by 45% if boys and 48% of girls. Coffee was consumed by 17% of both sexes. The majority of young people reported having milk as a drink although the proportion not drinking milk increased with age to 12-15% of 15- 18-year-olds. Semi-skimmed milk was the usual type of milk drunk by over a third of 4- 6-year-olds and over half those aged 11 and over.

Energy intakes

Mean intakes

Mean energy intakes were lower than estimated average requirements (EARs) for all age/sex groups, but were lowest in relation to the EARs for 15- 18-year-old girls. This may be partly due to under-reporting of food consumption in this group. Energy intakes in this survey were lower than in the 1983 survey of 10-11- and 14-15-year-old schoolchildren. However, young people in this survey were taller and heavier than in previous surveys, which suggests that their energy needs are lower.

Energy from fats

The average proportion of food energy derived from total fat was 35% for boys and 36% for girls, close to the COMA recommendation of 35%. The average proportion of food energy derived from saturated fatty acids was 14.2% for boys and 14.3% for girls, above the COMA recommendation of 11%.

Energy from sugars

Non-milk extrinsic sugars (NMES) provided on average 16.7% of food energy for boys and 16.4% for girls, which exceeded the COMA recommended average for the population of no more than 11%. The main source of NMES intake

---

Children's diets

The following poll found children's diets seriously short on fruit and vegetables

Q. 1 Which of the following vegetables do you like and hate the most?

	Like	Hate
Carrots	28%	3%
Sweetcorn	27%	3%
Peas	12%	6%
Broccoli	8%	8%
Cabbage	3%	4%
Cauliflower	3%	6%
Sprouts	3%	39%
Mange Tout	1%	3%
Courgette	1%	7%
Aubergine	*%	6%
I don't like/hate any of them	7%	6%
Don't know/not stated	6%	9%

Q. 2 Which of the following fruits do you like and hate the most?

	Like	Hate
Strawberry	33%	1%
Apple	18%	1%
Banana	10%	8%
Kiwi fruit	10%	10%
Mango	7%	4%
Peach	7%	2%
Tangerine	5%	2%
Plum	3%	4%
Tomato	1%	23%
Avocado	1%	22%
I don't like/hate any of them	1%	17%
Don't know/not stated	4%	5%

* denotes a finding of less than 0.5% but greater than zero

Source: MORI

was carbonated soft drinks, followed by chocolate confectionery.

Vitamin and mineral intakes
Average vitamin intakes
Average intakes of all vitamins except vitamin A were well above reference nutrient intakes (RNIs). Mean vitamin A intakes were close to or above the RNI in younger children but below the RNI in older groups. Up to a fifth of older girls and 12% of older boys had vitamin A intakes below the lower reference nutrient intake (LRNI) and a fifth of older girls had intakes of riboflavin below the LRNI. The main food sources of vitamin A were vegetables, providing about a quarter of average intake, and milk and milk products, providing about a fifth. The main sources of riboflavin were milk and milk products and cereals and cereal products (mainly fortified breakfast cereals), each providing about a third of average intake.

Average mineral intakes
Average intakes of most minerals in the youngest group were above the RNI, with the exception of zinc, and the percentage with intakes below the LRNI was small. However, in the older groups, average intakes for a number of minerals were below the RNI: zinc in all groups, potassium, magnesium and calcium in older boys and girls, and iron in older girls. Significant proportions of young people had intakes below the LRNI for some minerals.

Energy expenditure
Levels of physical activity
Information collected on the time that young people aged 7 and over spent in moderate or vigorous intensity activities indicates that most young people were inactive. The classification based on the calculated activity score suggests that activity levels were higher, but this is an over-estimate. Girls were less active than boys and activity levels fell with increasing age. About a third of 7- 14-year-old boys and over half the eldest boys failed to meet the HEA recommendation for young people to participate in at least moderate intensity activity for one hour a day. For girls, over half the 7-

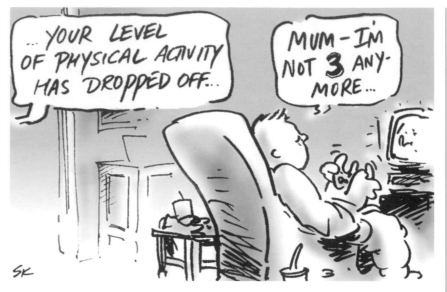

14-year-old group and over a third of the eldest group failed to meet this recommendation. There was no significant variation in physical activity levels with social class, region, household income or being at school or work. However, boys from families in receipt of benefits had significantly lower activity scores than other boys.

Transport into school
About 50% of young people walked to school, about one-third travelled by car and about 20% by bus. Between 1% and 6% cycled to school. Boys were significantly more likely to cycle to school than girls. Older children were significantly less likely to travel by car.

Physical measurements
Weight and height
Data on physical measurements showed that young people were taller and heavier than those studied in the 1982/3 survey of the Diets of British Schoolchildren. Boys were significantly taller and heavier than girls from the age of 16 years. Height and weight were positively associated with income.

Regional and socio-economic differences
Regional differences
Although there were some regional differences in diets there were few significant differences in energy and macronutrient intakes between regions. Intakes of most vitamins and minerals tended to be lower in Scotland, and to a lesser extent in Northern England, than elsewhere.

When differences in energy intakes were taken into account, lower intakes in Scotland persisted for vitamin D for boys and girls, iron and manganese for boys and thiamin, folate and pantothenic acid for girls and in Northern England for intakes of zinc for boys and girls and iron and manganese for girls. Young people in Scotland and the North also tended to have lower biochemical status of vitamins such as vitamin C and folate.

Socio-economic difference
Indicators of socio-economic status such as receipt of benefits, household income and social class showed that young people, particularly boys, in households of lower socio-economic status had lower intakes of energy, fat, some other macronutrients and most vitamins and minerals. Intakes of vitamin C, calcium, phosphorus, magnesium and iodine for boys and girls, pantothenic acid for boys and riboflavin, niacin, carotene and manganese for girls remained lower. Differences in energy intakes were taken into account, indicating differences in the quality of the diet between socio-economic groups for these nutrients. Those in lower socio-economic groups also tended to have lower biochemical status of vitamins such as folate, riboflavin, vitamin D and iron.

■ The above information is from the Advertising Association's web site which can be found at www.adassoc.org.uk
© The Advertising Association

Teen waistlines expanding

By Jenny Hope

Teenagers' bulging waistlines could leave them facing years of ill health, doctors have warned. Youngsters between 11 and 16 have the biggest waistlines ever recorded – up by more than two inches in ten years.

Body fat around the middle has been closely linked to life-threatening diseases.

Poor diets, sedentary lifestyles and the habit of slumping in front of the TV have created a generation who are piling on pounds that could lead them to an early death

Four times as many children are obese today compared with the 1980s and almost one in five is overweight, according to doctors.

Poor diets, sedentary lifestyles and the habit of slumping in front of the TV have created a generation who are piling on pounds that could lead them to an early death.

A report in the *British Medical Journal* says the most worrying statistic is the increasing size of the teenage waist.

Researcher Dr David McCarthy said waist measurements gave a much more accurate estimate of the number of fat children than simply comparing weight and height. 'We are in the middle of an obesity epidemic affecting our children,' he said.

'We already knew that having more upper body fat increases the risk for adults of heart disease and diabetes and it is a great cause for concern that for the first time we can see how much children's waistlines are expanding.

'It is very worrying because this is not just puppy fat – this is a population shift affecting children of all ages.'

A study by Dr McCarthy and colleagues at London Metropolitan University looked at data collected on the height, weight and waist circumference of 4,560 children between 11 and 16.

It found a rise in waist size of 2.5 ins between the mid-1980s and 1997 for both boys and girls. At 11, girls measure 25.5 ins on average around the waist and boys are 27ins. At 16, the average girl's waist is 29ins and boys measure 32ins.

Researchers found 39 per cent of girls and 28 per cent of boys were overweight, compared with 9 per cent for both a decade ago

Using waist circumference as a guide, the researchers found 39 per cent of girls and 28 per cent of boys were overweight, compared with 9 per cent for both a decade ago.

Dr McCarthy hopes to develop a set of 'ideal' waistline measurements to help parents work out if their children are at risk. Although there has been a fall in calories consumed by children, they are leading less active lives, he said.

© The Daily Mail

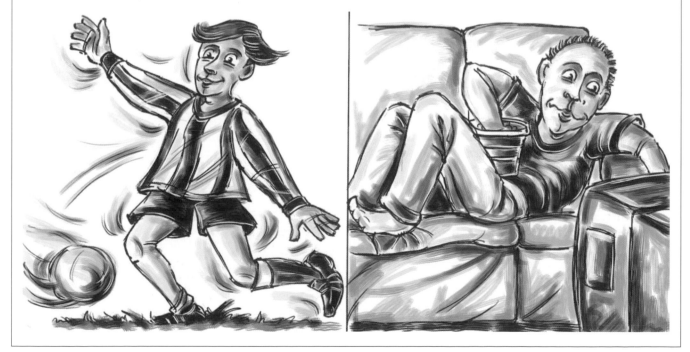

UK faces child diabetes epidemic

Obesity and lack of exercise to blame

By Jo Revill, Health Editor

Britain is facing an epidemic of diabetes among children and teenagers within a decade because of soaring rates of obesity and lack of exercise.

Medical experts have warned that poor nutrition in the first few years of life, low levels of physical activity and genetic factors are combining to leave a generation with unprecedented health problems.

If left unchecked, they predict that the cost of obesity-related diabetes care will swallow up the extra billions of pounds earmarked by the Chancellor for the NHS. There are currently around 100 teenagers with the condition, but this is predicted to rise tenfold within the next seven years. By 2020, thousands of teenagers are expected to have the condition, which can lead to damaged arteries and eyesight.

> *Around one in five adults in Britain is now overweight, and 9 per cent of boys and 13 per cent of girls between the ages of five and 16 are classified as obese*

Last year, the first white teenagers in Britain were diagnosed with Type II diabetes, previously only seen in adults and teenagers from Asian families where there was a genetic predisposition to the disease. There are now younger children showing signs of glucose intolerance, often a precursor to diabetes, who are being treated by specialists in London.

The Type II condition develops when the body can still make some of the hormone insulin but not enough, or when the insulin that is produced does not work properly (known as insulin resistance). Insulin helps the cells take in fuel in the form of blood sugar, but if the glucose doesn't reach the cells it builds up in the bloodstream, causing damage to the blood vessels and organs.

This type of diabetes, sometimes known as adult-onset diabetes, usually appears in people over the age of 40, and can be treated by diet and exercise or through tablets, but there can be complications.

Around one in five adults in Britain is now overweight, and 9 per cent of boys and 13 per cent of girls between the ages of five and 16 are classified as obese. Although children are consuming fewer calories than in previous generations, the food is higher in fat, salt and sugar and they are not exercising enough.

Dr Tom Smith, a GP who is an expert in diabetes, said: 'Diabetes is one of the leading causes of premature death in the UK. Unless we wake up to the problems caused by obesity, we're going to see soaring rates of this condition. Schools should be looking at providing 10 hours of exercise a week. At the moment there are schools which aren't even offering one-fifth of that.'

> *The Government has pledged to try to reduce obesity rates, by setting up initiatives across Britain*

The Government has pledged to try to reduce obesity rates, by setting up initiatives across Britain to encourage people to adopt a healthier lifestyle. Sir Steve Redgrave, the rower who was diagnosed with the condition before the 2000 Sydney Olympics, is fronting a campaign starting this week to find those who may unknowingly have impaired glucose intolerance.

And at a conference today doctors will highlight how the roots of obesity are laid down in the womb and childhood.

■ This article first appeared in *The Observer*, 8 June, 2003.
© Guardian Newspapers Limited 2003

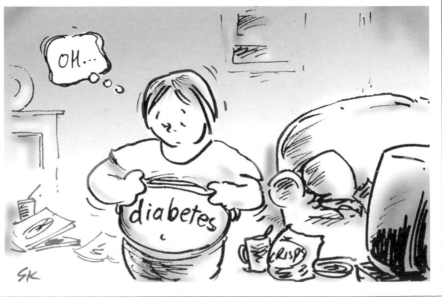

Obesity – defusing the health time bomb

It is well recognised that overweight and obesity increase the risk of this country's biggest killer diseases – coronary heart disease and cancer – as well as diabetes, high blood pressure and osteoarthritis. The National Audit Office (NAO) found that obesity is responsible for more than 9,000 premature deaths each year in England and reduces life expectancy on average by nine years. Obesity also has significant financial costs, both to the NHS and the wider economy. In common with other countries around the world, levels of obesity in England are rising. The consequences are serious.

Key points

Obesity levels in England have tripled in the past two decades; around a fifth (21%) of men and a quarter (24%) of women are now obese whilst almost 24 million adults are now overweight or obese. Obesity is also rising among children – in the five years between 1996 and 2001, the proportion of obese children aged 6-15 years rose by some 3.5. Cases of maturity-onset diabetes are starting to emerge in childhood. Worldwide, around 58% of type 2 diabetes, 21% of heart disease and between 8 and 42% of certain cancers are attributable to excess body fat. Obesity is responsible for 9,000 premature deaths each year in England, and reduces life expectancy by, on average, 9 years. Obesity costs the economy at least £2.5 billion a year – including costs to the NHS and cost to industry through sickness absence. Stemming the increase in obesity rates will need effective measures to improve diet and increase exercise levels in the population. Action by the food and fitness industries, as well as by government and local agencies, is needed.

The scale of the problem

The growth in the number of people in the population who are overweight

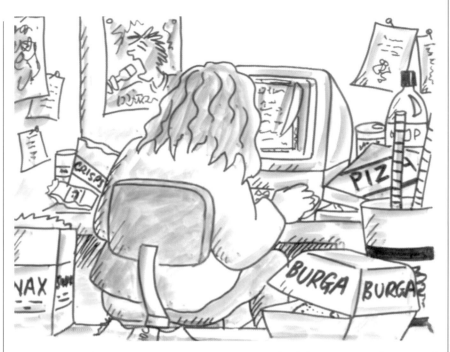

and obese is of increasing concern in most developed countries of the world. So much so that it has been termed a 'global epidemic'.

Overweight and obesity are most commonly assessed through the Body Mass Index (BMI) – calculated by dividing a person's weight in kilograms by their height in metres squared (kg/m^2). In England, an individual is considered to be 'overweight' if their BMI is between 25 and 30, and obese if over 30. Based on these definitions, around 21% of adult men and 24% of adult women are now obese. A further 47% of men and 33% of women are overweight. So, two-thirds of all men, and half of all women are now overweight or obese. This is almost 24 million adults. Rates have been rising in England, in common with other countries, and have trebled in the last 20 years.

Over the last few years in particular, public attention has been drawn by a number of influential bodies to the problem of obesity. This concern is not misplaced. Obesity rates have increased dramatically in most developed countries. Although levels of obesity in England have not yet reached those seen in the United States – where at the start of the 21st century almost a third (31%) of all adults are obese (an increase from a quarter just a decade earlier) – a continuation of the recent trend of rising numbers of overweight and obese people would be disastrous for the future health of our country. Globally now, more than one billion adults are overweight and at least 300 million are obese.

Children: a particular concern

Obesity is more common in older age groups but the growth in the proportion of overweight and obese children is a major concern. Analyses of the Health Survey for England suggest that a considerable number of children are either overweight or obese – for example, in 2001 8.5% of 6-year-olds and 15% of 15-year-olds were obese. Despite differences of view on the definition of overweight and obesity in childhood, all recent studies, no matter which method is used, have shown that overweight and obesity are becoming more common amongst children in England. Between 1996 and 2001 the proportion of overweight children (aged 6-15 years) increased by 7% and obese children by 3.5. Particularly worrying are the first signs of children presenting with maturity-onset (or type 2) diabetes which in the past has occurred in middle and older age. Researchers in the United Kingdom have recently warned that the increase in obesity threatens to reverse gains in longevity made during the last hundred years and in some cases could result in parents outliving their children.

A health inequalities issue

Obesity is also a health inequalities issue – and there are large social class differences, particularly in women. The Health Survey for England has shown that in 2001 amongst professional groups 14% of men and women are obese, compared to 28% of women and 19% of men in unskilled manual occupations. Amongst women, there are also important differences between ethnic groups: in 1999 obesity was 50% higher than the national average amongst Black Caribbean women and 25% higher amongst Pakistani women.

Health risks of obesity

As well as increasing mortality, it is well established that obesity is also associated with increasing the risk of many serious diseases.
Obesity is associated with increased risk of:
- Premature death
- Heart disease and stroke
- Type 2 diabetes
- Hypertension
- Angina

- Gall bladder diseases
- Osteoarthritis
- Sleep apnea
- Breathing problems
- Some cancers, including post-menopausal breast cancer and colon cancer
- Lower back pain
- Complications in pregnancy
- Complications in surgery
- Psychological and social problems
- Reproductive disorders

It is estimated that if no action is taken, globally we will see a one-third increase in the loss of healthy life as a result of overweight and obesity over the next 20 years

---

The rapid increase in obesity in the United States has also been mirrored by an increase in the prevalence of diabetes – by a third between 1990 and 1998. Such a scenario is also being seen here, where 75% of adults with newly diagnosed type 2 diabetes are overweight or obese. In 2002, cases of 'adult onset' diabetes in obese children were reported for the first time in the United Kingdom.

Implications

The World Health Organisation has recently highlighted that in 2002 alone, around half a million people across North America and Europe will die from obesity-related diseases. It is estimated that if no action is

taken, globally we will see a one-third increase in the loss of healthy life as a result of overweight and obesity over the next 20 years, with the number of global deaths rising from three million to five million each year. The World Health Organisation estimates that around 58% of type 2 diabetes, 21% of heart disease and between 8% and 42% of certain cancers are attributable to excess body fat.

For the NHS, it has been estimated that, based on current trends of increase, a general practice with 10,000 patients and five doctors would have to cope with 80 new obese patients each year. Already there is a significant increase in NHS costs. Since the National Institute of Clinical Excellence (NICE) issued guidance on the prescribing of the anti-obesity drugs Orlistat and Sibutramine in 2001, the number of these drugs dispensed has trebled.

For those who are already obese, even a modest weight loss can have substantial benefits. A 10kg loss is associated with a 20% fall in total mortality and a 10% reduction in total cholesterol. Based on the National Audit Office figures, it is estimated that one million fewer obese people in this country could lead to around 15,000 fewer people with coronary heart disease, 34,000 fewer people developing type 2 diabetes, and 99,000 fewer people with high blood pressure.

■ The above information is from the Chief Medical Officer's Health Report 2002.

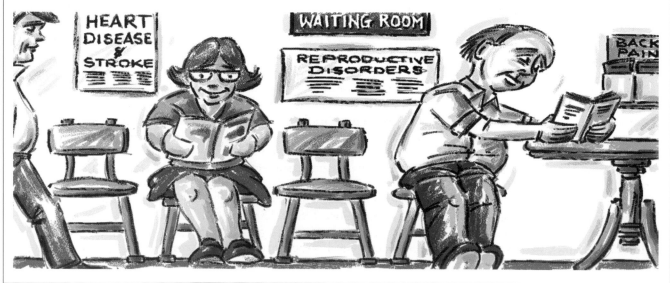

The trouble with girls

For many girls now sitting GCSEs, being bright and pretty is not enough: they have to be the brightest and the prettiest. What drives this obsessive perfectionism? And how dangerous is it?

By Oliver James

Last year Eleanor Kennedy scored four A-stars, four As and a B in GCSEs at her all-girl comprehensive school. You'd expect her to be overjoyed. Yet she shrugs and says: 'I wasn't pleased. All my friends did better. I felt terrible.'

Eleanor, 17, is at home in her west London sitting room with her friend, Jessica Wear. Jessica, also 17, thinks Eleanor is an 'idiot' because she 'did really well' – but she knows plenty of other girls who worry as much as Eleanor. 'I've one friend who's incredibly stressed-out, yet she got 10 A-stars. There's so much competition between girls in all ways now: how you look and dress, how clever you are, everything.'

Both girls appear fine to me, quick-wittedly fielding my questions and able to talk easily about their emotions. Sharp as a tack, Eleanor is perhaps naturally more of a worrier than Jessica but you wouldn't think either was an example of an alarming trend among teenage girls – girls like Charlotte, who goes to St Paul's Girls' School in London. She says she has felt 'anxious and depressed' since she was 13. 'I was obsessed with body image, always worrying about other people's opinions – whether they liked me or thought I was attractive'.

As teenage girls all over Britain prepare to sit their GCSEs, you would expect stress levels to be high. Yet this isn't ordinary exam anxiety. These middle-class, high-achieving girls are examples of a huge leap in rates of emotional disturbance among schoolgirls revealed in a groundbreaking study by Patrick West and Helen Sweeting of Glasgow University. They have discovered that, compared with only 16 years ago, young girls are dramatically – worryingly – more miserable.

West measured levels of anxiety and depression in two large, representative samples of 15-year-old children in 1987 and again in 1999.

Among the bottom social class, girls' rates rose only slightly – but in the top class the rise ranged from 24 per cent to a startling 38 per cent. Even more disturbing, West discovered that serious mental illness – the kind that can require hospitalisation – has risen threefold in middle-class teenage girls.

Mary Macleod, chief executive of the National Family and Parenting Institute, has noticed the trend: 'Professionals working with girls say the pressure to be beautiful, successful and popular is acute and damaging.' She adds that at this time of year exam hype is at such a pitch that some girls will find the stress too much and attempt to kill themselves.

Meanwhile, contrary to popular perceptions of a teenage male emotional apocalypse, researchers report no significant increase in problems among boys.

So what has happened? Why are girls at so much greater risk of severe emotional problems, despite having more opportunities than any generation before? Why do girls like Charlotte talk more about stress and self-hatred, depression and doubt, than what they're going to do with their friends on Saturday night?

West decided to ask the girls detailed questions about what made them so miserable. Schoolwork, exams, weight and family problems were mentioned most. What's fascinating is that the jump in anxiety levels exactly matches the time frame – between 1987 and 1999 – when girls began to outperform boys in almost every academic subject at every educational stage. In 1987 there was virtually no gender gap in GCSE performance. By 1999 53 per cent of girls were getting A-C grades at GCSE but only 43 per cent of boys were matching them.

West provides strong evidence that these girls find the period preceding exams more stressful than boys of any class or low-income girls, and that this difference has only arisen recently. And we're not just talking about teenagers immersed in the hot-house pressure of a highly academic private education: most of the girls in West's study attended comprehensive school.

Valerie Walkerdine, who did a small, in-depth study of high-achieving middle-class British girls in the Nineties, says: 'For the majority of middle-class girls high performance is regarded as average. A young woman who does well would not see herself as particularly outstanding because achievement was what was expected of her. By contrast, a working-class girl who does well would be held up as a good example by friends and family. The talents of middle-class achievers are largely unsung.'

These points should apply as much when comparing affluent boys with poor boys yet there seems to have been no change in the pressure on them to do well since 1987.

Joanna Kennedy, 52, a leading litigation lawyer and the mother of Eleanor, says: 'The pressure on girls to perform academically is far, far greater than when I was 15. I went to a convent, where very few girls would be expected to go to university. They really did say to us, "We are training you to be the wives of ambassadors". Even then I asked, "Why not to be the ambassador?"'

The greater vulnerability of girls to academic pressure may partly result from a greater desire to please. Joanna Kennedy remembers: 'Watching other parents when Eleanor was small, docility was prized in girls whereas it wasn't in boys at all. "That's a good girl" was awarded only to obedient, docile girls, from a very, very young age.'

Abundant scientific evidence suggests that repeated experiences of this kind early in life create a markedly greater tendency among girls to want to please authority and to be compliant. They become far more law-abiding as teenagers and adults, whether it be obedience to traffic regulations or committing fewer serious crimes. Above all, this people-pleasing makes them much more vulnerable to school cultures in which academic success is highly valued. Placed in a highly competitive GCSE school environment, it seems to be hard for girls to avoid worrying.

Jessica Wear recalls: 'The school put me under so much pressure. They used to say to me. "We've only had one B in the last five years – don't be the second." We were just – "aargh, how can we ever live up to that?"'

Eleanor Kennedy became part of an intensely competitive clique. 'I had genius friends and we'd work incredibly hard to be the cleverest. We'd predict who was going to get what score before a test. I used to get really upset when people got better marks than me.'

These kinds of cliques focusing on academic performance do not seem to be nearly as common among boys. Compare Charlotte, Eleanor, and Jessica with James Goldstone, 16, who attends Latymer School in London. He says: 'Boys are just less bothered about work. For GCSEs you're just regurgitating stuff you've been fed for two years. It's not that hard, and it is not very satisfying so you don't care if you get an A or an A-star – and you don't much care what other people get either.'

It may also be that parental pressure, specifically on daughters rather than sons, has increased. Joanna Kennedy says: 'You do see an awful lot of parents who are very anxious about their daughters' achievements. We went round one girls' school with Eleanor in mind and I thought that nothing would induce me to send her there because of the parents. You'd go to the chemistry lab and the fathers would be asking how many bunsen burners there were – incredibly intense anxiety.'

There seems to have been an outbreak of perfectionism among affluent daughters. The perfectionist feels her best is never good enough
---

There seems to have been an outbreak of perfectionism among affluent daughters. The perfectionist feels her best is never good enough. She sets impossibly high standards, rigidly imposed with a fanatical intolerance of mistakes. She has an intense fear of failure and is plagued by self-doubt. Even when she does achieve goals she feels dissatisfied, focusing on what she got wrong or belittling her success. Her main concern is to do better than others rather than the pleasure, in itself, of carrying out a task. Her self-esteem relies on winning, whether at work or play.

Such girls are prone to depression, despite their outward success, and to obsessive thoughts. Charlotte says: 'If I do something less than perfectly I will think about it for a long time. It's petty, but in my mock GCSEs I got two As, and A-stars in the rest. One of the As was in maths and I cried for so long. It was my best subject and I didn't get the top: "Why not?", I obsessed.'

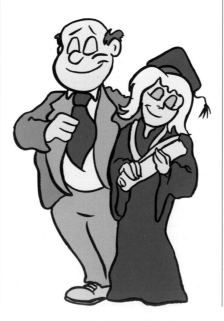

Girls like Charlotte are liable to have had perfectionist mothers from a generation that was frustrated by not being allowed to attend university. Discouraged from fulfilling their career potential, they poured these ambitions into their daughters rather than their sons because they identified with them more. In some cases this has simply righted the wrongs of previous generations – but it has also created many perfectionists.

Such mothers believe they only want the best for their daughter but in practice they tend to treat the girl as an agent for satisfying their own ambitions by making their love conditional on performance and by being excessively controlling. On top of that, the girl gets a double message: her mother is saying 'do well at school to get a high-flying career' – but when she looks at her as a role model she sees a full-time mother.

In other cases, where the mother is herself a high achiever, she may have high hopes for her daughter because of witnessing her own mother's lack of opportunity. Joanna Kennedy says: 'I was brought up by a mother who had no choices. I have this vision of a Fifties woman who was still economically dependent on a man. I wanted to encourage Eleanor to do well enough to have choices.'

Yet it would be unfair to heap all the blame on perfectionist mothers. For one thing, fathers now do one-third of childcare, so they may be contributing, although their impact tends to be more on boys than girls. (Girls' perfectionism is largely unaffected by their relationship with fathers.) For another, the care mothers provide is heavily influenced by social pressures and it only creates the potential for a problem; what happens in wider society determines whether that potential is fulfilled.

A crucial change from 1987 for affluent girls is the sheer number of criteria against which they now judge themselves. Eleanor's friend Jessica has noticed this: 'Girls try to have it all: be really clever, have a great social life and have lots of friends, and be pretty and thin. What leads to high stress is juggling all of them.'

Perhaps the greatest increase has been in concerns about weight, a major worry for affluent girls in West's study. It has become normal for young women to be irrationally critical of their bodies. In a 1998 British survey of 900 18- to 24-year-old women, more than half of those of average weight wished they could be slimmer; 40 per cent did not feel comfortable naked in front of their partners and 20 per cent said they stayed at home at least once a month because they were so dissatisfied with how they looked.

This is a problem for all girls, but girls from fee-paying schools are more at risk of eating disorders than those at state schools, and middle-class girls are more likely to want to be slimmer (whatever their actual weight) than less well-off ones.

Nancy, 16, another pupil at St Paul's, is of average weight for her height but tells me: 'I'd like to be thinner. Hardly anyone at school eats normally. You're always thinking other girls have better legs, better breasts, whatever.'

When Eleanor Kennedy was part of her GCSE clique, weight was also high on the list of criteria for comparative competition. 'It gets ridiculous – discussing what diets we should go on next week, what new forms of exercise to take up. I used to go to the gym for about three hours a day at one point.'

Interestingly, the problem was greatest among her 'genius friends'. 'My class were particularly foolish, and I knew a girl from another school who got 10 A-stars. She also happens to be the most beautiful girl in the world, perfect in every way, yet she was saying, "Oh, I need to go on a diet".'

This kind of comment is precisely what the studies predict: perfectionism, scholastic success and eating disorders often go together. In Charlotte's case it became a serious problem. She is back to a normal weight now but for a time she was bordering on the anorexic. 'I never felt like getting up in the mornings, tried to avoid mirrors. People told me I was underweight but I didn't believe them. I saw fat where others saw very thin.'

West's study also found a threefold increase in worries about weight among boys compared with 1987 – yet this was still less than half the girls' level. James Goldstone says: 'I do know a few perfectionist boys ... but we call them girls.'

The obsession with weight is almost certainly due to increased consumption of images of thin models and celebrities depicted in magazines and on television. There is strong evidence that these foster anxieties – indirectly through their effect on men's standards of what is attractive, as well as directly on women's.

On their own, these pressures would have stimulated girls' anxieties about weight, but it is no coincidence that they happened when there was also unprecedented pressure for girls to achieve academically. In a little-known series of studies American psychologist Brett Silverstein has shown that in periods when women are competing hotly with men academically and professionally, the Thin Standard (as measured by the ratio of bust and hip to waist measurements) is thinner. Hypothesising that for women to succeed in a man's world they might want to play down their femininity through slim androgyny, Silverstein showed that women who preferred smaller breasts and smaller buttocks were also more likely to choose 'masculine' careers and desire high academic achievement.

Like all doting parents I can bore for Britain about the creativity and zest for life of my 17-month-old daughter. The fascination that new objects evoke in her, the ebullience she brings to a seemingly common-place event, the living in the present . . . if only we adults could have bottled some of that joyfulness from our own childhoods.

It sickens me to think there is a serious risk this wonderful exuberance will give way to fearful concerns about schoolwork and her appearance in the eyes of others. I want her to succeed and to feel good about the way she looks – but not at any price.

■ Some names have been changed.

■ Oliver James is the author of *They F*** You Up – How to Survive Family Life* (Bloomsbury, £7.99). Patrick West and Helen Sweeting's study 'Fifteen, female and stressed' is published in the *Journal of Child Psychology and Psychiatry*, Volume 44.

■ This article first appeared in *The Observer*, 1 June 2003.

Girl talk

Every month I have coursework to submit and it's always a struggle to get it done. Teachers put more stress on me than my parents do. Sometimes I find myself up late, unable to sleep because I'm worried about getting everything done.
Zoe, 14

I've never been totally comfortable about my weight. I see women in the press and think, I'd love to be that thin, or have those legs. I'm pretty laid-back about exams but the coursework I find quite worrying. Sometimes I have been in a complete panic, really feeling low and not working effectively. I felt ill and couldn't do any work, I spend too much time filled with worry.
Katie, 17

My parents put quite a lot of pressure on me. They always expect the best. Neither of them went to university: my Dad was offered a place at Trinity College in Dublin and he didn't take it. He wanted to look after his family, things were different then. I suppose he wants me to take up his forfeited opportunity and succeed in that way.
Lisa, 17

It's pretty much a given that I will go to university. I work part time as well as doing my A-levels. I work between four and six hours a week, have done for about three years, and I find it difficult to sort out my time. That gets me all stressed out.
Caroline, 17

I put a lot of pressure on myself. I want to succeed at school and do well in life all round. I'm starting to look at universities now. Meanwhile, my brother's 22 and he still doesn't know what he wants to do.
Lara, 17

Interviews by Kirsty De Garis

Children's eating disorders

Children's eating disorders are toughest challenge for our counsellors, says new ChildLine report

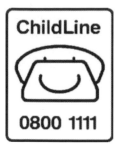

Helping young people battle an eating disorder is one of the toughest challenges ChildLine's counsellors face, according to a study of calls to the charity about the issue. Now a new report, *I'm in Control – Calls to ChildLine about eating disorders*, offers fresh insights into these life-threatening problems – revealing that friends are often the first to be told about a young person's eating disorder, and that family members have a vital part to play if a young sufferer is to recover. The report (based on analysis of calls to ChildLine between April 2001 and March 2002) also found that an eating disorder is almost always part of an 'intertwined knot of problems' – including family breakdown, bullying, bereavement, and in some cases abuse – which must be unravelled one by one before the process of recovery can begin.

Each year ChildLine helps around 1,000 children and young people suffering from eating disorders and last year almost 300 additional children spoke to the charity to seek advice about how to help a friend with an eating disorder. The report, sponsored by Next and written by award-winning journalist Brigid McConville, examines the gruelling and compelling testimony of young sufferers and demonstrates that there is rarely a single cause for an eating disorder.

ChildLine's Chief Executive, Carole Easton, says: 'This report makes a significant contribution to the debate on this difficult subject because it gives a voice to the young people whose lives are being destroyed by these debilitating conditions. We hope that it will form a springboard to greater understanding and offer fresh hope for young sufferers, as well as their friends and families. The pictures painted by this report are of intelligent, successful, high-achieving and determined young people who may seem unlikely to be vulnerable to destructive behaviours like anorexia and bulimia.

'However, a closer look often reveals a "knot of problems" out of which an eating disorder develops. Eating disorders may develop from a need for young people to feel a sense of control, to communicate feelings, and to block out painful emotions. All too often young people get a sense of self-worth from controlling their intake of food and this is what makes it so challenging for others to help break the iron grip of an eating disorder.

'Children and young people in their thousands turn to ChildLine's experienced counsellors every day of the year to talk about every problem imaginable – including those as harrowing as abuse, and attempted suicide. Yet our counsellors say that, of all the problems they help young people with, eating disorders are among the most challenging. This report shows that ChildLine's counsellors can help to cut through the confusion of denial and distortion facing loved ones when they try to help. When children call ChildLine and talk to a counsellor about an eating disorder they have already taken the first step along the difficult road to recovery – acknowledging that there is a problem. ChildLine is empowering for young people as they are in charge of the process and can call or write when they choose. The relationship can take on a special resonance as their counsellor can't see them and therefore can't "judge" them on their appearance.'

The report reveals that:

- Friends are enormously influential and have an important part to play in coping with an eating disorder. A significantly higher number of callers said they had told a friend (31%) rather than their mother (16%) or their GP (9%) about their illness. Friends are crucial in supporting each other, and are often extremely distressed by what their friend is going through – many call ChildLine to speak to a counsellor about the effect of an eating disorder on a friend.

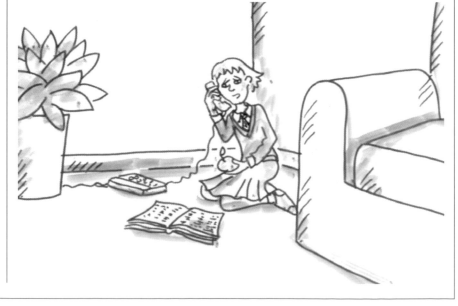

- For family and friends, helping a young person with an eating disorder can be incredibly difficult – yet young sufferers tell ChildLine that the support of people around them is indispensable. More than any other issue, family tensions are mentioned in conversations with young people about eating problems. A quarter of those who call ChildLine to talk primarily about an eating disorder also discuss family difficulties, including conflict between parents, resentment about siblings and an atmosphere of unhappiness and tension at home. However, in many cases it is unclear whether these difficulties were a precursor to the eating disorders or had arisen as a result. The report also shows that parents are extremely supportive and a crucial source of help to their children.
- Adolescence and the accompanying emergence of an adult sexual identity is often the time when a young person is most vulnerable to the onset of an eating disorder. Of callers who mentioned their age, three-quarters (74%) in ChildLine's sample were between the ages of 13 and 16. It is clear from the calls that children as young as 11 have a vocabulary that includes the words anorexia and bulimia. Children in the younger age group frequently talk about the physical symptoms of their eating disorder, while older callers are often the veterans of hospitals and clinics and have a deeper understanding of what they're going through.
- Young people tell ChildLine about a wide range of factors that they believe triggered their problem. These usually include a situation or event that threatens their self-identity or security or lowers their self-esteem. The circumstances most often mentioned by callers include family problems, bullying, school pressures, loss of a friend or family member, illness and abuse.
- Calls to ChildLine demonstrate a range of reasons for the progression of an eating disorder, once it has been triggered off.

Among these is an increasingly distorted perception of body image and a sense that they are helpless to stem the progress of the eating disorder as it is 'out of control'. Pervasive social and media pressures to be thin influence the determination of many to control their body shape, as does the continued sensation that feeling thin equates with feeling good.

- A small minority of calls in the sample were from boys – only 50 of the 1,067 total. The experiences boys have in developing eating disorders appear similar to those of girls but there are significant differences in the way boys and girls talk about their eating problems and some of the triggers setting them off. These appear to be centred on the roles and behaviours considered acceptable to boys in society. The report discloses that boys are twice as likely to say that bullying is part of their problem and are far more likely to confide in their doctor or their mother about an eating problem – perhaps due to fear of being bullied by their peers. Calls to ChildLine also portray boys as feeling an additional sense of shame about having what is seen as a 'girl's problem'.
- Boys talk about their eating disorders in a more factual, straightforward way, unlike girls who tend to start by saying they're worried about their weight, and then to gradually unravel their 'bundle of problems'. Boys focus on the health or medical reasons for being thin, rather than the aesthetic explanations girls give. Girls often tell ChildLine that they feel judged, and judge themselves, on how they look and they generally express more self-hatred than boys, which is mirrored in the way they speak

about their bodies. In contrast to boys, the report's author found that some girls also appear to be in a kind of 'anorexic club' where they all diet and starve themselves to be thin.

Carole Easton says: 'Eating disorders are a minefield for everyone affected by them. One of the saddest revelations in ChildLine's report is the sense among some sufferers that their eating disorder is a coping mechanism that stops them from "doing something worse" – and "as an alternative to suicide, is a familiar friend that keeps them alive". The cycle of denial and deceit, and frequently withdrawn and angry behaviour of a young person with an eating disorder, can almost seem designed to drive away those who care about them, leaving parents and friends utterly bewildered and at a loss as to how to move forward.

'But our report also brings home the fact that friends and family must not give up – their love and support is essential in building up a young person's self-esteem and bringing them back to health. Although there is no single solution to the tortuous situation an eating disorder can provoke, families and friends are the best allies a young person has, and the most effective remedy is when everyone – friends, family, school, professionals, and ChildLine counsellors – works together to ensure there is always someone to turn to.'

Case studies

All identifying details have been changed

Becky, 14, called ChildLine because she wanted to know more about the symptoms of anorexia and bulimia. 'I've lost a lot of weight recently', she said. 'I only eat one meal a day and often I throw it up.' Becky told her counsellor that she enjoyed swimming at school but often felt faint when she did it. 'I've no energy so I've stopped doing exercise', she said. 'I haven't told my mum – we argue a lot.' Becky said she often felt fat – even though really she knew she wasn't.

Rhiannon, 13, was very upset when she called ChildLine. 'I got a swimsuit for my birthday but when I

'Eating disorders are a minefield for everyone affected by them'

---

tried it on I realised I'm too fat to wear it', she said. 'I know I'm fat because my friends at school tease me about it.' Rhiannon paused and then she said, 'I've started making myself sick. It's been a few months now.' She said she had done this in the past and had lost weight – but she had ended up in hospital. 'I liked being thin – but I didn't have any energy so I couldn't play out with my friends.' Rhiannon said that her mum always tried to make sure she ate regularly.

When Ian, 13, called ChildLine he said he had recently started a special diet to help him lose weight. Ian told ChildLine that he had been 'really overweight' so his GP had given him a course of medicine to suppress his appetite. 'They worked and I lost weight which made me happy', he said. Now that he had finished the course Ian told the counsellor that he felt 'very alone'

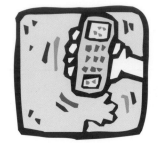

without the back-up of the drugs. 'Now I'm scared that if I start eating again I'll put the weight back on.' Since stopping taking the tablets he had only been 'snacking now and then'.

'My boyfriend is really annoying me', said 16-year-old Emma when she called ChildLine. 'He keeps asking me what I've had to eat – I always read the information on food to check I am eating well.' Emma told ChildLine that she was feeling pressured about her eating habits by several people in her life. 'My friends at school like pointing out who in

the group has put weight on and where on their body. And sometimes my dad says to me watch what you eat or you'll end up as big as your auntie.'

When Natalie, 15, called ChildLine she said, 'I want to talk about food. I can't stand the thought of it inside me – so I throw it up.' Natalie said she was very unhappy about her weight but couldn't talk to her family. 'I'm being picked on at school 'cause I'm fat. If my folks find out I may as well just run away – I think they're embarrassed to know me anyhow.' She said that she had always had a problem with her weight. 'I'm so big it's unreal', Natalie said. 'I feel like food is destroying me – making me feel bigger – but then I feel so hungry.'

■ The above information is from ChildLine's web site which can be found at www.childline.org.uk

© *ChildLine*

Young people and suicide

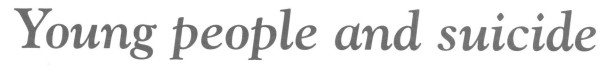

Information from the Samaritans

Last year, the rate of suicide amongst under-25-year-olds in the UK and Republic of Ireland remained constant at more than two per day in 2001.

The suicide rate amongst young men (15-24 years) in the UK has increased since the 1970s. However, in the UK and Ireland, the rate per 100, 000 in 2001 has continued on its five-year downward trend (from a five-year high of 18 per 100,000 in 1998) to 15 per 100,000, a level not seen before the early 1990s. This compares with an overall suicide rate in the general population of 12 per 100,000. In the Republic of Ireland, suicide amongst young men rose in the 1990s; between 1990 and the year 2000, the rate of 26 per 100,000 was an increase over that period of 73%. However, in 2001 this rate showed a substantial fall to a rate of 22 per 100,000. The rate amongst young men in Scotland, which stood at 36 per 100,000 in 2000, has shown a substantial fall to stand at 30 per 100,000 in 2001.

Amongst the factors linked to suicide and self-harm

Alcohol and drug abuse
Substance abuse is thought to be a highly significant factor in youth suicide. Alcohol and drugs affect thinking and reasoning ability and can act as depressants. They decrease inhibitions, increasing the likelihood of a depressed young person making a suicide attempt. American research has shown that one in three adolescents are intoxicated at the time of death, and a further number are under the influence of drugs. A recent Samaritans' study found that suicidal young men are 10 times more likely to use a drug to relieve stress.

Families
In general, adolescents who attempt to take their own lives appear to grow up in families with more turmoil than other groups of adolescents, coming more often from broken homes (due to death or divorce), homes where there is parental

unemployment, mental illness, or addiction.

Physical and sexual abuse
Young people who suffer, or have suffered, abuse in the past are often at increased risk of suicide or deliberate self-harm. General violence has also been found to play an extensive role in the lives of suicidal young people when compared with the non-suicidal.

Custody
Within the prison population as a whole, young prisoners represent the largest group of at-risk individuals, particularly those under 21 who make up a substantial proportion of the remand population. In 2002, 27% of prison suicides were by people aged 15-20.

■ The above information is from the Samaritans' *Information Resource Pack 2003*. For more details visit their web site at www.samaritans.org.uk

© *Samaritans*

Youth and self-harm

Perspectives. A summary of research commissioned by the Samaritans and carried out by the Centre for Suicide Research, University of Oxford

Results

- 10 per cent of teenagers aged 15 and 16 years old have deliberately self-harmed – seven per cent in the previous year.
- The majority, more than 64 per cent, of those who self-harm cut themselves.
- Girls are nearly four times more likely to self-harm than boys.
- The most common reason given was 'to find relief from a terrible situation', the least common reason was 'to get my own back'.
- 41 per cent of those who self-harm seek help from friends before acting.

How common is self-harm?

Of the pupils surveyed 10.3 per cent carried out an act of deliberate self-harm (6.9 per cent in the previous year and 2.5 per cent in the previous month).

A unique aspect of this study was that the researchers asked the pupils to describe acts of self-harm rather than merely report whether or not they had ever harmed themselves. This enabled the researchers to accurately assess the acts of self-harm against set criteria.

Although this approach may have under-estimated the true numbers of those self-harming, as not all those surveyed supplied a

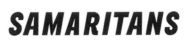

SAMARITANS

description, it does provide a more accurate picture than most research where participants are simply asked whether or not they have self-harmed.

What methods do young people use to self-harm?

Just 12.6 per cent of the incidents of self-harm described by pupils in the survey resulted in a hospital visit. This may be explained by the preference of those who self-harm to cut rather than poison themselves: poisoning is more likely to end in hospital than minor self-cutting. The results of the research showed that

---

Of the pupils surveyed 10.3 per cent carried out an act of deliberate self-harm (6.9 per cent in the previous year and 2.5 per cent in the previous month).

---

some 64.6 per cent of those that had self-harmed in the previous year had cut themselves compared to 31.7 per cent who poisoned. Other not so frequently used methods of self-harm included self-battery, use of recreational drugs, use of alcohol, hanging or suffocation.

Who is likely to self-harm?

The pupils most likely to self-harm were female – of those that had self-harmed in the previous year 11.1 per cent were female and just 3.2 per cent male. Female pupils were also more likely to have had suicidal thoughts – 22.4 per cent female compared to 8.5 per cent male.

Deliberate self-harm and suicidal thoughts were also more common among white and other, often mixed race, pupils than those from Black or Asian backgrounds.

Why does it happen?

The most common reasons given by pupils for deliberate self-harm were 'to find relief from a terrible state of mind' or because they had 'wanted to die'. Contrary to popular belief few were 'trying to frighten someone' or simply 'get attention'.

Who do they turn to for help?

Some 40.8 per cent of those who self-harmed had sought help from friends before hurting themselves. The results of the research showed that few turned to other sources of help such as family, teachers, doctors or social workers. Help was sought after the event by 22.1 per cent of those who self-harmed – 49 per cent of these received help from friends and 21 per cent from family.

What differentiates those who self-harm or have suicidal thoughts from those who do not?

- Those who self-harm have more problems and life events than other teenagers.

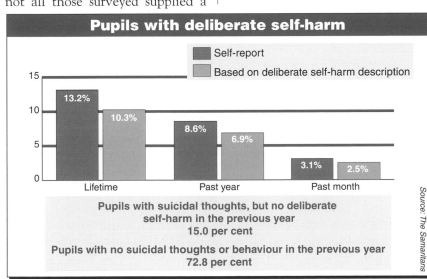

Pupils with deliberate self-harm

- Self-report
- Based on deliberate self-harm description

Lifetime: 13.2% / 10.3%
Past year: 8.6% / 6.9%
Past month: 3.1% / 2.5%

Pupils with suicidal thoughts, but no deliberate self-harm in the previous year
15.0 per cent

Pupils with no suicidal thoughts or behaviour in the previous year
72.8 per cent

Source: The Samaritans

- People who self-harm are also more likely to suffer anxiety, depression and have low self-esteem than others.
- Those that self-harm often have friends who self-harm.
- Girls who self-harm may have concerns about sexuality, boys may have suffered physical abuse.
- Those who self-harm find it difficult to cope and are more likely to blame themselves, get angry, drink alcohol or shut themselves in their room than talk things through.
- Those who self-harm believe they have fewer people in whom they can confide compared to other adolescents.

More 'life' problems

The teenagers were asked to report life events and problems encountered in the previous year such as boyfriend or girlfriend problems, death of a close relative, and physical abuse.

The results showed that those who deliberately self-harmed had experienced more problems in the previous year than those who reported suicidal thoughts. And those with suicidal thoughts had experienced more problems than those with neither deliberate self-harm nor suicidal thoughts.

The most common problems faced by all pupils were related to schoolwork. Also rating highly were problems with parents and having friends who self-harmed.

More anxiety and depression

In addition to being asked about life problems, the teenagers were asked about their current levels of anxiety, depression, impulsivity and self-esteem. The results showed that those pupils who reported self-harm or having suicidal thoughts were more likely to be suffering from anxiety and depression, were more impulsive and had lower self-esteem than those who did not.

More friends who have suicidal thoughts or self-harm

They were also more likely to have friends who self-harm or have suicidal thoughts – a common phenomenon which in the past has led to clusters

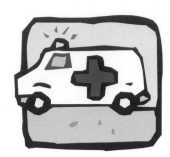

of teenage suicides, but which has not until now been explicitly linked to self-harming behaviour.

Poorer coping strategies

The research also showed, for the first time, that those who self-harmed were less able to cope when they felt worried or upset. Instead of using positive coping strategies, such as talking to someone or trying to sort out the situation, they were more likely to resort to negative strategies such as blaming themselves, getting angry, staying in their room or drinking alcohol.

Apart from friends – consulted by 85 per cent of all those surveyed – those who self-harmed or had suicidal thoughts had far fewer people in whom they felt able to confide.

Fewer people they can talk to

Those who self-harmed had fewer people with whom they felt able to talk about problems compared to other teenagers. Apart from friends – consulted by 85 per cent of all those surveyed – those who self-harmed or had suicidal thoughts had far fewer people in whom they felt able to confide. The majority of young people who self-harmed knew up to two people in whom they could confide, those with suicidal thoughts knew three, while those who neither self-harmed nor had suicidal thoughts had up to seven people in whom they could confide.

Differences between suicidal thoughts and self-harming behaviour

The results of the research found that some circumstances were found to be associated with either self-harm or suicidal thoughts but not both. These not only varied by circumstance, but by gender.

For instance, a family history of suicidal behaviour and drug use by the pupil were associated with self-harm but not suicidal thoughts.

For the female pupils, smoking and worries about sexual orientation led to suicidal thoughts but not self-harm – an issue which has previously received little attention. For the male pupils, physical abuse was a potential trigger for suicidal thinking.

Suicidal thoughts and self-harm

	Suicidal thoughts Males	Females	Deliberate self-harm Males	Females
Having friends who have engaged in suicidal behaviour	✔	✔	✔	✔
Family member had engaged in suicidal behaviour	✗	✗	✔	✔
Smoking	✗	✔	✗	✗
Drug use	✗	✗	✔	✔
Drunkenness in the previous year	✔	✔	✗	✗
Sexual orientation	✗	✔	✗	✗
Physical abuse	✔	✗	✗	✗
Depression	✗	✗	✗	✔
Anxiety	✔	✔	✗	✔
Low self-esteem	✔	✔	✔	✔
Impulsivity	✗	✗	✗	✔

Source: The Samaritans

Who do they turn to?

For all teenagers, teachers were the least likely source of comfort. Just 20.5 per cent of pupils felt that they could talk to a teacher, despite problems with schoolwork being closely associated with an increased likelihood of self-harm. Since young people clearly saw their friends as their key sources of support, it raises questions about whether they are able to recognise when friends are in trouble and if so, would be able to help.

Too embarrassed to seek professional help

Telephone helplines and professional organisations were often not contacted because adolescents said they were too embarrassed, didn't have the confidence, thought their problems were too trivial, or worried about confidentiality.

Ways in which they felt that organisations like Samaritans could be made more approachable included: giving advice rather than simply listening, advertising more to young people, recruiting younger people as volunteers, and making more school visits.

Conclusions

In summary, those who self-harm are likely to:

- Be female
- Be white
- Use cutting rather than poisoning
- Be looking for a way out of a situation rather than attention-seeking
- Have low self-esteem, anxiety or depression
- Be unable to cope effectively with problems
- Have worries about school work
- Have friends or family who self-harm
- Prefer to seek help from friends than relatives or teachers

The findings show that deliberate self-harm and suicidal thoughts are important problems in adolescence. They also provide a clear insight into how prevention and support for those at risk might be organised.

Educational programmes

Since the vast majority of pupils who

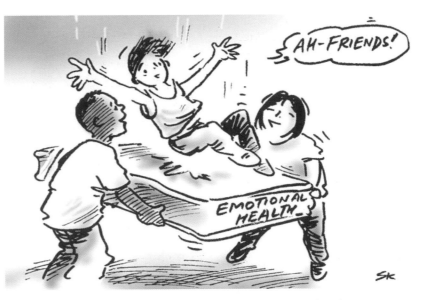

self-harm do not go to hospital, prevention needs to take place in the community, ideally within schools.

One possible approach is the development of educational programmes to promote psychological well-being, for example by helping pupils to recognise and deal with emotional problems.

As adolescents turn to their friends for help and advice, they will need help not only coping with their own emotional problems but also in recognising and helping friends in need.

Teachers might also be helped to recognise pupils who are getting into difficulties. A more controversial approach that might be considered is the use of screening in schools to detect those pupils at risk.

Whichever approach is adopted, schools will need advice on what to do when self-harm is recognised – especially if a cluster of acts seems to be developing. This clearly has implications for teacher training.

Schools will also need the support of other professionals, including health, social services and voluntary organisations. With this in mind it will be important to talk to pupils and find out exactly how they would like help delivered.

Next steps: the role of Samaritans

Recognising that young people need to know more about what help is available and advice on caring for their own well-being,

Samaritans is developing an emotional health promotion strategy. This will aim to encourage young people to recognise the value of being able to express feelings and to respect and acknowledge the feelings of others.

Samaritans' Emotional Health Promotion Programme will be rolled out in 2003-2004. As part of this programme, young people in schools will be presented with more effective coping and help-seeking strategies. Samaritans is also working with other organisations, including YouthNet UK, that specifically offer advice to young people.

A fresh approach

The research also clearly shows that young people feel there is a stigma attached to approaching voluntary organisations. Samaritans has recently changed its approach to young people – promoting itself in new ways including an email helpline. Meanwhile, Samaritans is targeting its recruitment campaigns to attract volunteers who are younger and who belong to a variety of minority groups.

By using the results of this research, it is hoped that pupils, schools and voluntary services can help young people to cope with emotional problems without resorting to self-harm.

■ The above information is from the Samaritans' web site which can be found at www.samaritans.org.uk

© Samaritans

- Most students in the 1997/1998 survey consider themselves healthy (total 91.8%, range 81.2% to 98.0%). By a small but consistent difference, a higher percentage of males (93.7%) than females (90.0%) report feeling very healthy; and this pattern is consistent for all countries and regions. (p. 1)

- The vast majority of students report feeling happy (85.2%, 62.2% and 94.1% of 11- 13- and 15-year-olds, respectively). (p. 2)

- The overall percentage of students feeling low on a weekly basis is relatively high, averaging over 25%. (p. 2)

- There is evidence that patterns of health behaviours established in adolescence are maintained through adult life (e.g. smoking, substance abuse, eating disorders, physical activity, obesity and sexual risk taking). (p. 4)

- Regular physical activity provides young people with important physical, mental and social health benefits. (p. 5)

- Adolescence may be defined as the process of growing up. The age span is variable as young people mature at different ages and speeds. The World Health Organization puts the ages between 11 and 21. (p. 6)

- Under-age drinking and problems associated with it are increasing in the UK. Surveys show that children drink alcohol earlier, and by their teens, drinking is a regular part of their lives. Between 92% and 98% of 15-years-olds have tried alcohol. (p. 7)

- Children starting to smoke at the age of 15 years are three times more likely to die from smoking than adults starting in their mid twenties. (p. 7)

- Experimental substance abuse is common in early adolescence, but only a minority will eventually develop addictive patterns of use. (p. 9)

- One youngster in every 14 has sex in their first teenage year, research has revealed. (p. 10)

- One in four girls is reported to have had sex before the age of 16 and one in 12 has asked for contraception at a sex clinic at the age of 14. (p. 10)

- The UK has the highest rate of teenage pregnancies in western Europe. (p. 11)

- The age at which the majority of 16-19-year-olds today first have sexual intercourse is 16. Almost 30% of young men and almost 26% of young women report having intercourse before their 16th birthday. (p. 13)

- In 2001, 29% of pupils reported that they had ever tried one or more drugs, 20% had taken drugs in the last year and 12% had done so in the last month. (p. 14)

- Levels of alcohol abuse by children have almost doubled over the past ten years. (p. 16)

- Overall, 18 per cent of pupils aged 11 to 15 said they had taken drugs in the previous 12 months. (p. 16)

- A total of 28 per cent of pupils said they have been offered cannabis. (p. 16)

- More teenage girls are taking up smoking just to keep their weight down, evidence suggests. (p. 17)

- Children who smoke are two to six times more susceptible to coughs and increased phlegm, wheeziness and shortness of breath than those who do not smoke. (p. 18)

- There has been a big increase in 'binge drinking' among children and young people, with almost a third of 15- and 16-year-olds drinking more than five drinks on a single occasion in the last week – an increase of nearly 50 per cent over eight years. (p. 21)

- A comparative European study of drinking among 15-16-year-olds (ESPAD) showed that UK figures for alcohol consumption were some of the highest in Europe alongside Ireland and Denmark. (p. 23)

- Boys are more likely than girls to do exercise because it makes them healthy (56% compared to 48%), while girls are likely to do exercise to look good and lose weight (11% compared to 4%). (p. 24)

- Four times as many children are obese today compared with the 1980s and almost one in five is overweight, according to doctors. (p. 27)

- Around one in five adults in Britain is now overweight, and 9 per cent of boys and 13 per cent of girls between the ages of five and 16 are classified as obese. (p. 28)

- It is estimated that if no action is taken, globally we will see a one-third increase in the loss of healthy life as a result of overweight and obesity over the next 20 years. (p. 30)

- Each year ChildLine helps around 1,000 children and young people suffering from eating disorders and last year almost 300 additional children spoke to the charity to seek advice about how to help a friend with an eating disorder. (p. 34)

- The suicide rate amongst young men (15-24 years) in the UK has increased since the 1970s. However, in the UK and Ireland, the rate per 100, 000 in 2001 has continued on its five-year downward trend. (p. 36)

- Substance abuse is thought to be a highly significant factor in youth suicide. Alcohol and drugs affect thinking and reasoning ability and can act as depressants. (p. 36)

- Girls are nearly four times more likely to self-harm than boys. (p. 37)

ADDITIONAL RESOURCES

You might like to contact the following organisations for further information. Due to the increasing cost of postage, many organisations cannot respond to enquiries unless they receive a stamped, addressed envelope.

The Advertising Association
Abford House
15 Wilton Road
London, SW1V 1NJ
Tel: 020 7828 2771
Fax: 020 7931 0376
E-mail: aa@adassoc.org.uk
Web site: www.adassoc.org.uk
The Advertising Association is a federation of 25 trade bodies representing the advertising and promotional marketing industries including advertisers, agencies, media and support services. It is the only body that speaks for all sides of an industry that was worth over £16.7 billion in 2002.

Alcohol Concern
Waterbridge House
32-36 Loman Street
London, SE1 0EE
Tel: 020 7928 7377
Fax: 020 7928 4644
E-mail: contact@alcoholconcern.org.uk
Web site: www.alcoholconcern.org.uk
Alcohol Concern aims to develop more and better treatment services nationally, to increased public and professional awareness of alcohol misuse and to bring about a reduction in alcohol-related problems.

Alcohol Education and Research Council (AERC)
Room 408, Horseferry House
Dean Ryle Street
London, SW1P 2AW
Tel: 020 7217 8028
E-mail: info@aerc.org.uk
Web site: www.aerc.org.uk
The Council was established by the Government in 1982 by an Act of Parliament (The Licensing (Alcohol Education and Research Act 1981) to administer the Alcohol Education and Research Fund. This Fund finances projects within the United Kingdom for education and research and for novel forms of help to those with drinking problems.

ASH – Action on Smoking and Health
102 Clifton Street
London, EC2A 4HW
Tel: 020 7739 5902
Fax: 020 7613 0531
E-mail: enquiries@ash.org.uk
Web site: www.ash.org.uk
Tobacco is unique: the only product that kills when used normally – 120,000 deaths per year in the UK. ASH is leading the fight to control the tobacco epidemic and to confront the tobacco industry.

Brook Advisory Centres
Unit 421, Highgate Studios
53-79 Highgate Road
London, NW5 1TL
Tel: 020 7284 6040
Fax: 020 7284 6050
E-mail: admin@brookcentres.org.uk
Web site: www.brook.org.uk
Brook Advisory Centres – commonly known just as Brook – is the only national voluntary sector provider of free and confidential sexual health advice and services specifically for young people under 25. If you need to speak to someone urgently, you can call the Brook Helpline on 0800 0185 023.

ChildLine
45 Folgate Street
London, E1 6GL
Tel: 020 7650 3200
Fax: 020 7650 3201
E-mail: reception@childline.org.uk
Web site: www.childline.org.uk
ChildLine is a free, national helpline for children and young people in trouble or danger. Provides confidential phone counselling service for any child with any problem 24 hours a day. Children or young people can phone or write free of charge about problems of any kind to: ChildLine, Freepost 1111, London N1 0BR, Tel: Freephone 0800 1111.

Health Development Agency (HDA)
Holborn Gate
330 High Holborn
London, WC1V 7BA
Tel: 020 7430 0850
Fax: 0207 413 8900
Web site: www.hda.nhs.uk
HDA identifies the evidence of what works to improve people's health and reduce health inequalities. In partnership with professionals, policy makers and practitioners, it develops guidance and works across sectors to get evidence into practice.

Royal College of Paediatrics and Child Health
50 Hallam Street
London, W1W 6DE
Tel: 020 7307 5600
E-mail: enquiries@rcpch.ac.uk
Web site: www.rcpch.ac.uk
The aim of the association from the very beginning was the advancement of the study of paediatrics and the promotion of friendship amongst paediatricians.

The Samaritans
The Upper Mill
Kingston Road, Ewell
Surrey, KT17 2AF
Tel: 020 8394 8300
Fax: 020 8394 8301
E-mail: jo@samaritans.org.uk
Web site: www.samaritans.org.uk
Deals with suicide-related issues. Their help line is open 24 hours a day: 08457 90 90 90

World Health Organization (WHO)
20 Avenue Appia
1211-Geneva 27
Switzerland
Tel: + 41 22 791 2111
Fax: + 41 22 791 3111
E-mail: info@who.ch
Web site: www.who.int
WHO works to make a difference in the lives of the world's people by enhancing both life expectancy and health expectancy.

ACKNOWLEDGEMENTS

The publisher is grateful for permission to reproduce the following material.

While every care has been taken to trace and acknowledge copyright, the publisher tenders its apology for any accidental infringement or where copyright has proved untraceable. The publisher would be pleased to come to a suitable arrangement in any such case with the rightful owner.

Chapter One: Overview

Adolescents' general health and wellbeing, © World Health Organization (WHO), *Low and lonely*, © World Health Organization (WHO), *Young people have major health needs*, © Royal College of Paediatrics and Child Health, *Physical activity and youth*, © World Health Organization (WHO), *Young adults*, © 2002 Elsevier Ltd., *Young people's health*, © 2002 Elsevier Ltd., *The state of young people's health in the EU*, © European Commission.

Chapter Two: Issues in Adolescent Health

Teenage sex shock, © The Daily Mail, *Teenage pregnancy and parenthood*, © Health Development Agency (HDA), *Teenage sexual activity*, © Brook Advisory Centres, *Drug use among young people*, © Crown copyright is reproduced with the permission of Her Majesty's Stationery Office, *Young people and drugs*, © Crown copyright is reproduced with the permission of Her Majesty's Stationery Office, *One in three teens 'has smoked cannabis'*, © The Daily Mail, *Models 'drive girls to smoke'*, © The Daily Mail, *Young people and smoking*, © ASH, *Smoking*, © ASH, *Conspicuous consumption*, © 0-19 Magazine, *Alcohol sales to underage adolescents*, © Alcohol Education and Research Council (AERC), *Alcohol sales*, © Alcohol Education and Research Council (AERC), *Young people's drinking*, © Alcohol Concern, *UK youth too busy to 'get physical'*, © 2003 MORI, *Diet and nutrition*, © The Advertising Association, *Children's diets*, © 2003 MORI, *Teen waistlines expanding*, © The Daily Mail, *UK faces child diabetes epidemic*, © Guardian Newspapers Limited 2003, *Obesity – defusing the health time bomb*, © Crown copyright is reproduced with the permission of Her Majesty's Stationery Office, *The trouble with girls*, © Guardian Newspapers Limited 2003, *Children's eating disorders*, © ChildLine, *Young people and suicide*, © The Samaritans, *Youth and self-harm*, © The Samaritans, *Pupils with deliberate self-harm*, © The Samaritans, *Suicidal thoughts and self-harm*, © The Samaritans.

Photographs and illustrations:

Pages 1, 9, 27, 30: Pumpkin House; pages 4, 12, 20, 29, 34: Bev Aisbett; pages 5, 10, 14, 17, 19, 21, 28, 39: Simon Kneebone.

Craig Donnellan
Cambridge
September, 2003